Sergio Arturo Galindo-Rodríguez

Aspects pharmaceutiques des nanoparticules polymériques

Sergio Arturo Galindo-Rodríguez

Aspects pharmaceutiques des nanoparticules polymériques

Formulation et transposition d´échelle

Presses Académiques Francophones

Impressum / Mentions légales
Bibliografische Information der Deutschen Nationalbibliothek: Die Deutsche Nationalbibliothek verzeichnet diese Publikation in der Deutschen Nationalbibliografie; detaillierte bibliografische Daten sind im Internet über http://dnb.d-nb.de abrufbar.
Alle in diesem Buch genannten Marken und Produktnamen unterliegen warenzeichen-, marken- oder patentrechtlichem Schutz bzw. sind Warenzeichen oder eingetragene Warenzeichen der jeweiligen Inhaber. Die Wiedergabe von Marken, Produktnamen, Gebrauchsnamen, Handelsnamen, Warenbezeichnungen u.s.w. in diesem Werk berechtigt auch ohne besondere Kennzeichnung nicht zu der Annahme, dass solche Namen im Sinne der Warenzeichen- und Markenschutzgesetzgebung als frei zu betrachten wären und daher von jedermann benutzt werden dürften.

Information bibliographique publiée par la Deutsche Nationalbibliothek: La Deutsche Nationalbibliothek inscrit cette publication à la Deutsche Nationalbibliografie; des données bibliographiques détaillées sont disponibles sur internet à l'adresse http://dnb.d-nb.de.
Toutes marques et noms de produits mentionnés dans ce livre demeurent sous la protection des marques, des marques déposées et des brevets, et sont des marques ou des marques déposées de leurs détenteurs respectifs. L'utilisation des marques, noms de produits, noms communs, noms commerciaux, descriptions de produits, etc, même sans qu'ils soient mentionnés de façon particulière dans ce livre ne signifie en aucune façon que ces noms peuvent être utilisés sans restriction à l'égard de la législation pour la protection des marques et des marques déposées et pourraient donc être utilisés par quiconque.

Coverbild / Photo de couverture: www.ingimage.com

Verlag / Editeur:
Presses Académiques Francophones
ist ein Imprint der / est une marque déposée de
AV Akademikerverlag GmbH & Co. KG
Heinrich-Böcking-Str. 6-8, 66121 Saarbrücken, Deutschland / Allemagne
Email: info@presses-academiques.com

Herstellung: siehe letzte Seite /
Impression: voir la dernière page
ISBN: 978-3-8381-7481-5

TABLE DES MATIÈRES

I

AVANT-PROPOS

Ces dernières années, de nombreuses études se sont focalisées sur le développement de nanoparticules de polymères en tant que systèmes d'administration de substances médicamenteuses. En effet, ces systèmes colloïdaux possèdent des caractéristiques physico-chimiques permettant la libération contrôlée ou ciblée de molécules actives. En fonction de leur taille (10-1000 nm), les nanoparticules peuvent traverser les membranes biologiques, être transportées dans les capillaires sanguins les plus fins (5-6 µm de diamètre) et subir une absorption cellulaire. De plus, la grande surface spécifique de ces colloïdes leur permet, d'une part, d'établir un contact intime avec leur substrat biologique (organe, tissu ou cellule), et d'autre part, d'associer des ligands spécifiques (invasines, lectines et anticorps) propres à induire un ciblage actif. Finalement, l'état solide des ces vecteurs protége le principe actif encapsulé de la dégradation lors de son transport dans l'organisme.

Il existe un grand choix de techniques de préparation des nanoparticules, ce qui représente un avantage important du point de vue technologique et pharmaceutique. En effet, selon la méthode de fabrication :

i)   il est possible d'incorporer des principes actifs hydrophiles ou hydrophobes, ainsi que des molécules biologiques (protéines, peptides et oligonucléotides);

ii) des polymères aux propriétés très variables peuvent être utilisés permettant ainsi la modulation du comportement biologique des ces vecteurs (bioadhésion, biodégradation, biocompatibilité, bioreconnaissance) et la libération de la molécule active; et

iii) finalement, les caractéristiques physiques des nanoparticules telles que leur taille, structure, morphologie et surface (rugosité et charge) peuvent être aussi modifiées.

Les avantages et les inconvénients liés à chacune des méthodes de préparation de nanoparticules ont été fréquemment reportés. Cependant, des études comparatives de ces techniques font généralement défaut. Les informations issues de telles études paraissent de grande utilité car on pourrait établir des règles de formulation en vue de choisir la méthode la plus appropriée pour la fabrication des nanoparticules de propriétés préalablement définies.

En conséquence, pour ce travail de thèse nous avons sélectionné trois des techniques les plus utilisées pour la préparation de nanoparticules, et les avons comparées en termes de leurs différents paramètres pharmaceutiques et technologiques. Les techniques retenues incluent deux méthodes de fabrication partant d'une émulsion (relargage ou *salting-out* et émulsification-diffusion) ainsi que la nanoprécipitation. Dans ce contexte, le premier chapitre présente une brève revue bibliographique de ces techniques. Dans le deuxième chapitre, les performances de ces techniques ont été évaluées en fonction de leur capacité d'incorporer dans les nanoparticules un principe actif légèrement soluble dans l'eau, l'ibuprofène. Le troisième chapitre donne une approche technologique propre à transférer ces trois techniques à une échelle pilote. Dans le quatrième chapitre, nous reportons l'encapsulation de deux molécules possédant une activité anticancéreuse ainsi que l'évaluation biologique des nanoparticules obtenues. Enfin, le dernier chapitre comprend une revue de la littérature sur les diverses études consacrées à l'application *in vivo* des nanoparticules par la voie orale.

III

CHAPITRE I

TECHNIQUES DE PRÉPARATION DE NANOPARTICULES À BASE DE POLYMÈRES

TECHNIQUES DE PRÉPARATION DE NANOPARTICULES À BASE DE POLYMÈRES

S. Galindo-Rodríguez, E. Allémann, E. Doelker and H. Fessi

Over the past few decades, there has been considerable interest in the use of polymeric nanoparticles as potential drug delivery systems. These colloidal carriers may offer some advantages such as protection of drugs against degradation, targeting of drugs to specific sites of action (organ or tissue), and delivery of biological molecules such as proteins, peptides and oligonucleotides. Depending on their composition and intended use, they can be administered orally, parenterally, or locally [1-4].

The advantages conferred by these colloidal carriers for use in drug delivery result from their physicochemical characteristics: sub-micron size, large specific surface area, versatile surface properties (e.g. hydrophobicity, charge) and variable polymer composition. First, their small size enables nanoparticles to cross biological membranes, be transported through the smaller capillaries (5-6 μm in diameter) and be taken up by cells, which allows efficient drug accumulation at target sites. Second, the large specific surface area of nanoparticles ensures an intimate contact between the colloidal carrier and the biological substrate (e.g. tissues or cells) as well as the possibility for the incorporation of specific ligands (e.g. invasins, lectins and antibodies) for inducing active targeting. The modulation of their surface properties enables alteration of certain biological phenomena such as biorecognition, biodistribution, bioadhesion and cellular uptake. Finally, by changing their

2

composition, for instance using biodegradable materials, nanoparticles offer an extended release of the encapsulated drug within the target site over a period of days or even weeks.

Numerous methods exist for the manufacturing of nanoparticles, allowing extensive modulation of their physicochemical properties. The choice of the manufacturing method essentially depends on the raw material used (e.g. polymer) and on the solubility characteristics of the active compound to be associated to the nanoparticles. With respect to the raw material, criteria such as biocompability, degradation behavior, choice of the administration route, desired release profile of the drug, and finally the type of biomedical application determine its selection. Basically, the preparation methods employed must include the following requirements:

i) The stability and biological activity of the drug should not be altered during the encapsulation process.

ii) The yield of nanoparticles having the required size range and drug encapsulation efficiency should be high.

iii) The nanoparticle quality and the drug release profile should be reproducible within specified limits.

iv) The nanoparticles should be produced as redispersible powder and should not exhibit aggregation or adherence.

Practically, nanoparticles have been prepared mainly by two methods: i) dispersion of the preformed polymers and ii) polymerization of monomers [1,3,5,6].

Various authors have reported the preparation of nanoparticles by polymerization of monomers [1,7-9]. For instance, nanoparticles of about 200 nm can be obtained by polymerizing the dispersed methyl or ethyl cyanoacrylate in an aqueous acidic medium in the presence of polysorbate 20 as a surfactant. Briefly, the cyanoacrylate monomer is added to an aqueous solution of the surface-active agent under vigorous mechanical stirring to polymerize alkylcyanoacrylate at ambient temperature. The drug is dissolved in the polymerization medium either before the addition of the monomer or at the end of the polymerization reaction. The suspension of nanoparticles is then purified by ultracentrifugation or filtration. During polymerization, various stabilizers such as dextran and poloxamer are added.

Particle size and molecular mass of nanoparticles depend upon the type and concentration of the stabilizer and surfactant used, and the pH of the polymerization medium [10-12]. Other factors include the concentration of monomer and the stirring rate [11,13]. Nanoparticles from poly(methylmethacrylate) and related copolymers are also prepared by polymerization of monomers [14-16]. Recently, Bouchemal et al. developed a technique involving interfacial polycondensation combined with spontaneous emulsification for producing nanocapsules from poly(urethane) and poly(ether urethane) [9]. The preparation of nanoparticles by polymerization still suffers from shortcomings. First, because of the multicomponent nature of the polymerization media, it is generally very difficult to predict the molecular weight of the resulting polymerized material. This is a major drawback because the molecular weight greatly influences the release behavior of the polymeric carrier. Another limitation is related to the presence of toxic residues such as the unreacted monomer and the initiator, whose elimination is complicated. Finally, the polymerization reaction could induce the degradation or inactivation of the drug [3,6].

The main methods for preparing nanoparticles from preformed polymers can be classified into four categories: nanoprecipitation, emulsification-evaporation, salting-out, and emulsification-diffusion. The common feature of these techniques is that they involve an organic solution containing the components of nanoparticles that functions as an internal phase during preparation, and an aqueous solution containing stabilizers that constitutes the dispersion medium of the nanoparticles. The last three techniques are also known as emulsion-based methods since their procedures require the preparation of an emulsion. Figure 1 shows the general procedure for manufacturing nanoparticles from preformed polymers. Other methods developed for manufacturing nanoparticles from preformed polymers, which will not be discussed in this paper, are the phase inversion encapsulation [17], double emulsion [18-22] and supercritical fluid spraying [23,24] techniques (Table I).

The method of nanoprecipitation was developed and patented by Fessi and co-workers [25,26]. This technique involves the use of an organic solvent that is completely miscible (e.g. acetone, ethanol or methanol) with the aqueous phase. It allows the preparation of nanospheres as well as nanocapsules without prior emulsification. Briefly, the polymer, drug and optionally a lipophilic stabilizer (e.g. phospholipids) are dissolved in the water-miscible solvent. This solution is

5

poured or injected into an aqueous solution containing a stabilizer (e.g. poly(vinyl alcohol) or poloxamer 188) under magnetic agitation. Nanospheres are formed instantaneously by rapid solvent diffusion, which is then eliminated from the suspension under reduced pressure. The incorporation of an oily compound (e.g. Miglyol® N812) into the organic phase allows the preparation of nanocapsules [26,27].

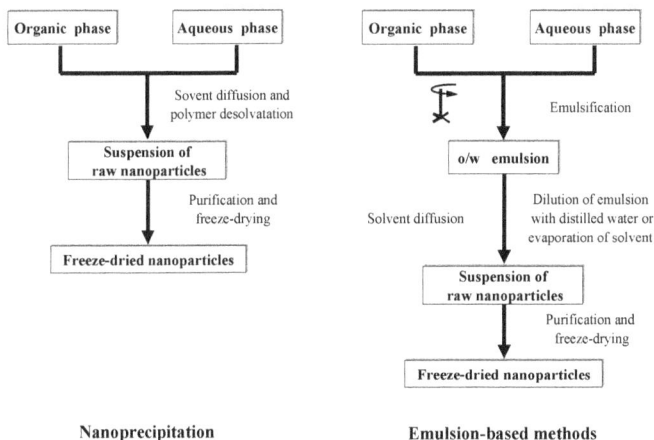

Figure 1. Manufacturing of nanoparticles from preformed polymers by the nanoprecipitation technique and the emulsion-based methods (emulsification-evaporation, salting-out and emulsification-diffusion).

For the nanoprecipitation method, the mean size and recovery of nanoparticles have been shown to be significantly affected by the concentration of polymer [28]. This behavior was attributed to an increase in the viscosity of the organic phase. In addition, it seems that the concentration of stabilizers in the aqueous phase has a minor influence on the mean size of nanoparticles.

The usefulness of the nanoprecipitation technique is limited to drugs that are highly soluble in polar organic solvents, but only slightly soluble in water. In general, this method has to be carried out with low concentrations of polymer in the organic phase allowing polymer dispersion and a small particle size to be obtained easily. In contrast, when it is necessary to increase the amount of polymer in the organic phase, large aggregates tend to form, resulting in poor productions yields.

Emulsification-evaporation is a well established method based on the classical procedure patented by Vanderhoff and co-workers [29]. The preformed polymer and the drug are dissolved in a water-immiscible or partially water-immiscible organic solvent such as dichloromethane, chloroform or ethyl acetate. Subsequently, an o/w emulsion is obtained by adding the organic phase to an aqueous phase containing an emulsifying agent (e.g. gelatin, poly(vinyl alcohol), polysorbate 80, poloxamer 188). This crude emulsion is then exposed to a high energy-source such as an ultrasonic device or is passed through homogenizers, colloid mills, or microfluidizers to reduce the size of the globules. The subsequent evaporation of the organic solvent, either by increasing the temperature under pressure or by continuous stirring at room temperature, results in the formation of a fine aqueous dispersion of nanospheres.

For this technique, two main process parameters are considered relevant: i) the homogenization step which allows the formation of particles with a submicron size, and ii) the evaporation step which influences the internal structure of nanoparticles (e.g. porosity) as well as their drug loading. A very rapid solvent evaporation may cause local liquid/gas transitions inside the droplets and lead to

7

formation of porous structures on the particle surface. Basically, the rate of solvent evaporation depends on the vapor pressure of the solvent as well as on the temperature and pressure during evaporation.

The salting-out procedure was patented by Bindschaedler et al. in the late eighties [30]. This method is based on the separation of a water-miscible solvent from aqueous solution via a salting-out effect. This technique makes use of acetone instead of the chlorinated solvents used in the emulsification-solvent evaporation method. The preparation method consists of dissolving polymer and drug in the organic solvent. Then, the organic phase is emulsified under mechanical stirring in an aqueous solution containing an electrolyte as the salting-out agent and a colloidal stabilizer. Subsequently, the oil-in-water emulsion is diluted with a sufficient volume of water to induce the diffusion of acetone into the external phase, thus leading to polymer precipitation in the form of nanospheres.

Several important factors influence the size of nanoparticles. By increasing the poly(vinyl alcohol) concentration in the external phase of the emulsion, a decrease in particle size is observed . An increase in the stirring rate and a decrease in the polymer concentration of the organic phase can also induce a reduction of particle size [28,31,32]. To achieve high drug loadings with this method, high solubility of the drug in acetone is required. Moreover, the selection of the salting-out agent is important because it can play an important role in the drug entrapment efficiency. For instance, it was reported that entrapment efficiency of savoxepin (pK_a = 8.3) can be significantly improved by using a basic salt (e.g. magnesium acetate) instead of neutral or acid salts [33]. The main advantage of the salting-out technique is the excellent yields of nanoparticles that can be obtained. However, the presence of salt in the aqueous phase represents the major limitation of this technique because the electrolyte can induce instability of some compounds including the drug and stabilizing agent. In addition, a purification stage of the raw dispersion of nanoparticles is always necessary in order to eliminate the high amounts of emulsifying agent and electrolyte.

The method of emulsification-diffusion is derived from the salting-out procedure and overcomes the problem of using large amounts of salt in the aqueous phase. This technique is based on the use of a partially water-soluble solvent (e.g. benzyl alcohol, propylene carbonate or ethyl acetate) [34-37]. First, the solvent and water are mutually saturated in order to ensure their initial thermodynamic equilibrium. Then, polymer and drug are dissolved in the organic solvent and the resulting solution is emulsified, under vigorous agitation, into an aqueous phase containing a stabilizing agent. The subsequent addition of water to the system induces the diffusion of the solvent into the external phase, resulting in the formation of nanoparticles. The polymer concentration in the organic phase, the internal phase-external phase ratio as well as the type and concentration of stabilizing agent in the aqueous phase are the main variables that influence the mean size of nanoparticles.

This technique presents some advantages over the other methods described above, such as the use of pharmaceutically acceptable organic solvents, lack of a homogenization step and high yields generally obtained. In addition, the preparation of nanospheres as well as nanocapsules is possible. For the particular case of nanocapsules, the thickness of the polymeric wall can be controlled by varying the polymer concentration in the organic phase. Two drawbacks can be mentioned for this technique: the high volume of water to be eliminated from the suspension of nanoparticles and the leakage of water-soluble drugs into the external phase during the solvent-diffusion step.

The wide choice of techniques for preparing nanoparticles represents an important advantage from the technological and pharmaceutical point of views (Table I). First, hydrophilic and hydrophobic drugs as well as biological macromolecules can be incorporated into the nanoparticles. Second, these nanoparticulate systems can be prepared using different polymeric materials which allow modulation of certain properties including the drug release rate, biodegradation and bioadhesion. Polymers used for this end can be of either natural (e.g. gelatin, chitosan, sodium alginate) or synthetic origin (e.g. poly(alkylcyanoacrylates), poly(lactic acid), poly(lactic-*co*-glycolic acid), poly[ethylene glycol-*co*-(lactic-glycolic acid)], poly(ε-caprolactone) and poly[methylmethacrylate]) [1,38-41]. Finally, physicochemical properties of these carriers such as size, internal structure and surface properties (e.g. roughness, zeta potential), can also be modified by using different preparation methods.

The methods for manufacturing nanoparticles have been often studied individually. Most studies have been focused on the process parameters of each technique that affect drug entrapment and particle size. However, very few studies exist in which the performance of these techniques are compared. Comparative studies are important to identify the most appropriate technique for preparing nanoparticles with specific characteristics in terms of size, drug loading, surface properties and yield.

Table I Methods for manufacturing polymeric nanoparticles.

Method	Polymer	Solvent system	Stabilizer	Nanoparticles size (nm)	Reference
Polymerization	PIBCA	—	Pluronic F68	160 – 190	[42]
	PECA	—	Pluronic F108	300 – 630	[43]
	PMMA / PMMA–PSPM	—		60 – 280	[14]
	PU / PEU	Acetone / Isopropyl alcohol	Span® 85 / Tween® 20	150 – 500	[9]
Nanoprecipitation	PLA / PLGA / PCL	Acetone	Pluronic F68	110 – 208	[44]
	PLGA	Acetone–ethanol / Acetone–methanol	PVAL	~ 260	[45]
	PCL	Acetone–ethanol	Pluronic F68	190 – 300	[42]
	PLGA	Acetonitrile		157 – 210	[46]
Emulsification–evaporation	PLA–PEG–PLA	Dichloromethane	PVAL	193 – 335	[47]
	PEO–PLGA	Methylene chloride	PVAL	~ 150	[48]
	PLA / PLGA / PLA–PEG	Methylene chloride	Sodium cholate / Albumin	150	[49]
	PLGA	Dichloromethane	PVAL	800	[50]

11

Method	Polymer	Solvent	Stabilizer	Size (nm)	Ref.
Salting-out	PLA	Acetone	PVAL	300 – 700	[51]
	PLA / PLGA	Acetone / Tetrahydrofuran	PVAL	100 – 350	[32]
	Eudragit® L100-55	Acetone	PVAL	108 – 710	[28]
Emulsification–diffusion	PLA / Eudragit® S100	Benzyl alcohol	PVAL / Gelatin	70 – 1350	[34]
	PLA	Propylene carbonate	PVAL / Poloxamer 188	130 – 1350	[35]
	Cellulose acetate phthalate	2–butanone	Poloxamer 407	400 – 3000	[37]
	Eudragit® E	Ethyl acetate	PVAL	390 – 1900	[37]
Double emulsion	PLA	Methylene chloride	PVAL / Albumin	190 – 285	[21]
	PLGA	Ethyl acetate	PVAL / Poloxamer 188	320 – 514	[52]
	PLA / PLA–PEG	Ethyl acetate	——	~ 160	[53]
	PLGA	Ethyl acetate / Methylene chloride	PVAL	335 – 743	[54]
Phase inversion nanoencapsulation	PLGA	Methylene chloride	——	> 5000	[17]

PIBCA, poly(isobutylcyanoacrylate); PECA, poly(ethylcyanoacrylate); PMMA, poly(methylmethacrylate); PMMA–PSPM, poly(methylmethacrylate-*co*-sulfopropylmethacrylate); PU, poly(urethane); PEU, poly(ether urethane); PLA, poly(lactic acid); PLGA, poly(lactic-*co*-glycolic acid); PCL, poly(ε-caprolactone); PVAL, poly(vinyl alcohol); PLA–PEG–PLA, poly(lactic acid)–poly(ethylene glycol)–poly(lactic acid); PEO–PLGA, poly[ethylene oxide-*co*-(lactic-glycolic acid)]; PLA–PEG, poly(lactic acid-*co*-ethylene glycol).

Therefore, the present study was aimed at comparing, from the pharmaceutical and technological points of view, the versatility of three of the most common methods used for manufacturing nanoparticles. The studied techniques include two emulsion-based methods (salting-out and emulsification-diffusion) and the nanoprecipitation procedure. First, the physicochemical parameters associated with the formation of nanoparticles by each technique were investigated. Second, the process parameters of each method that influence the incorporation of a slightly water-soluble drug (e.g. ibuprofen) into the nanoparticles were examined. Third, the feasibility of these techniques to produce nanoparticles on a pilot-scale was evaluated. Finally, the advantages and limitations of these procedures were determined for each stage of this study. Likewise, different physicochemical models were applied in order to describe the physicochemical phenomena associated with the formation and production of the polymeric nanoparticles.

Chapitre I

References

[1] P. Couvreur, G. Barratt, E. Fattal, P. Legrand, C. Vauthier, Nanocapsule technology: a review, Crit. Rev. Ther. Drug Carrier Syst. 19 (2002) 99-134.

[2] S. Davis, Biomedical applications of particle engineering, in: R. H. R. Coombs, W. D. Robinson (Eds.), Nanotechnology in Medicine and the Biosciences, Gordon & Breach, Amsterdam, Netherlands, 1st ed., 1996, pp. 243-262.

[3] F. De Jaeghere, E. Doelker, R. Gurny, Nanoparticles, in: E. Mathiowitz (Ed.), Encyclopedia of Controlled Drug Delivery, John Wiley, U. S. A., 1st ed., 1999, pp. 641-664.

[4] S. M. Moghimi, A. C. Hunter, J. C. Murray, Long-circulating and target-specific nanoparticles: theory to practice, Pharmacol. Rev. 53 (2001) 283-318.

[5] E. Allémann, R. Gurny, J. C. Leroux, Biodegradable nanoparticles of poly(lactic acid) and poly(lactic-co-glycolic acid) for parenteral administration, in: A. H. Lieberman, M. M. Rieger, S. G. Banker (Eds.), Pharmaceutical Dosage Forms: Disperse Systems, Marcel Dekker, Inc., 2nd ed., 1989, pp. 163-193.

[6] D. Quintanar-Guerrero, E. Allémann, H. Fessi, E. Doelker, Preparation techniques and mechanisms of formation of biodegradable nanoparticles from preformed polymers, Drug Dev. Ind. Pharm. 24 (1998) 1113-1128.

[7] P. Couvreur, B. Kante, M. Roland, et al., Polycyanoacrylate nanocapsules as potential lysosomotropic carriers: Preparation, morphological and sorptive properties, J. Pharm. Pharmacol. 31 (1979) 331-332.

[8] P. Couvreur, M. Roland, P. Speiser, Biodegradable submicronic particles containing a biologically active substances and compositions containing them, U.S. Patent 4 329 332, 1982.

[9] K. Bouchemal, S. Briancon, E. Perrier, H. Fessi, I. Bonnet, N. Zydowicz, Synthesis and characterization of polyurethane and poly(ether urethane) nanocapsules using a new technique of interfacial polycondensation combined to spontaneous emulsification, Int. J. Pharm. 269 (2004) 89-100.

[10] N. Behan, C. Birkinshaw, N. Clarke, A study of the factors affecting the formation of poly (n-butyl cyanoacrylate) nanoparticles, Proceedings of the Controlled Release Society (1999) pp. 1134-1135.

Techniques de préparation de nanoparticules à base de polymères

[11] N. Behan, C. Birkinshaw, N. Clarke, Poly n-butyl cyanoacrylate nanoparticles: a mechanistic study of polymerisation and particle formation, Biomaterials 22 (2001) 1335-1344.

[12] P. A. McCarron, A. D. Woolfson, S. M. Keating, Response surface methodology as a predictive tool for determining the effects of preparation conditions on the physicochemical properties of poly(isobutylcyanoacrylate) nanoparticles, Int. J. Pharm. 193 (1999) 37-47.

[13] R. Gaspar, V. Preat, M. Roland, Nanoparticles of polyisohexylcyanoacrylate (PIHCA) as carriers of primaquine: formulation, physico-chemical characterization and acute toxicity, Int. J. Pharm. 68 (1991) 111-119.

[14] K. Langer, C. Marburger, A. Berthold, J. Kreuter, F. Stieneker, Methylmethacrylate sulfopropylmethacrylate copolymer nanoparticles for drug delivery. Part I: Preparation and physicochemical characterization, Int. J. Pharm. 137 (1996) 67-74.

[15] F. Hoffmann, J. Cinatl, H. Kabickova, J. Cinatl, J. Kreuter, F. Stieneker, Preparation, characterization and cytotoxicity of methylmethacrylate copolymer nanoparticles with a permanent positive surface charge, Int. J. Pharm. 157 (1997) 189-198.

[16] H.-P. Zobel, A. Zimmer, S. Atmaca-Abdel Aziz, M. Gilbert, D. Werner, C. R. Noe, J. Kreuter, F. Stieneker, Evaluation of aminoalkylmethacrylate nanoparticles as colloidal drug carrier systems. Part I: synthesis of monomers, dependence of the physical properties on the polymerization methods, Eur. J. Pharm. Biopharm. 47 (1999) 203-213.

[17] G. P. Carino, J. S. Jacob, E. Mathiowitz, Nanosphere based oral insulin delivery, J. Control. Release 65 (2000) 261-269.

[18] A. Vila, H. Gill, O. McCallion, M. J. Alonso, Transport of PLA-PEG particles across the nasal mucosa: effect of particle size and PEG coating density, J. Control. Release 98 (2004) 231-244.

[19] F. Delie, M. Berton, E. Allemann, R. Gurny, Comparison of two methods of encapsulation of an oligonucleotide into poly(D,L-lactic acid) particles, Int. J. Pharm. 214 (2001) 25-30.

[20] M. F. Zambaux, F. Bonneaux, R. Gref, E. Dellacherie, C. Vigneron, Preparation and characterization of protein C-loaded PLA nanoparticles, J. Control. Release 60 (1999) 179-188.

Chapitre I

[21] M. F. Zambaux, F. Bonneaux, R. Gref, P. Maincent, E. Dellacherie, M. J. Alonso, P. Labrude, C. Vigneron, Influence of experimental parameters on the characteristics of poly(lactic acid) nanoparticles prepared by a double emulsion method, J. Control. Release 50 (1998) 31-40.

[22] A. Vila, A. Sanchez, M. Tobio, P. Calvo, M. J. Alonso, Design of biodegradable particles for protein delivery, J. Control. Release 78 (2002) 15-24.

[23] T. W. Randolph, A. D. Randolph, M. Mebes, S. Yeung, Sub-micrometer-sized biodegradable particles of poly(L-lactic acid) via the gas antisolvent spray precipitation process, Biotechnol. Prog. 9 (1993) 429-435.

[24] U. B. Kompella, K. Koushik, Preparation of drug delivery systems using supercritical fluid technology, Crit. Rev. Ther. Drug Carrier Syst. 18 (2001) 173-199.

[25] H. Fessi, J. P. Devissaguet, F. Puisieux, C. Thies, Procédé de préparation de systèmes colloïdaux dispersibles d'une substance, sous forme de nanoparticules, French Patent 2 608 988, 1986.

[26] H. Fessi, F. Puisieux, J. P. Devissaguet, N. Ammoury, S. Benita, Nanocapsule formation by interfacial polymer deposition following solvent displacement, Int. J. Pharm. 55 (1989) R1-R4.

[27] P. Legrand, G. Barratt, V. Mosqueira, H. Fessi, J. P. Devissaguet, Polymeric nanocapsules as drug delivery systems, S. T. P. Pharma Sciences 9 (1999) 411-418.

[28] S. Galindo-Rodríguez, E. Allémann, H. Fessi, E. Doelker, Physicochemical parameters associated with nanoparticle formation in the salting-out, emulsification-diffusion, and nanoprecipitation methods, Pharm. Res. 21 (2004) 1428-1439.

[29] J. W. Vanderhoff, M. S. El-Aasser, J. Ugelstad, Polymer emulsification process, U.S. Patent 4 177 177, 1979.

[30] C. Bindschaedler, R. Gurny, E. Doelker, Process for preparing a powder of water-insoluble polymer which can be redispersed in a liquid phase, the resulting powder and utilization thereof, U.S. Patent 4 968 350, 1990.

[31] E. Allémann, R. Gurny, E. Doelker, Preparation of aqueous polymeric nanodispersions by a reversible salting-out process: influence of process parameters on particle size, Int. J. Pharm. 87 (1992) 247-253.

[32] Y. N. Konan, R. Gurny, E. Allémann, Preparation and characterization of sterile and freeze-dried sub-200 nm nanoparticles, Int. J. Pharm. 233 (2002) 239-252.

Techniques de préparation de nanoparticules à base de polymères

[33] E. Allémann, J. C. Leroux, R. Gurny, E. Doelker, *In vitro* extended-release properties of drug-loaded poly(D,L-lactic acid) nanoparticles produced by a salting-out procedure, Pharm. Res. 10 (1993) 1732-1737.

[34] J. C. Leroux, E. Allémann, E. Doelker, R. Gurny, New approach for the preparation of nanoparticles by an emulsification-diffusion method, Eur. J. Pharm. Biopharm. 41 (1995) 14-18.

[35] D. Quintanar-Guerrero, H. Fessi, E. Allémann, E. Doelker, Influence of stabilizing agents and preparative variables on the formation of poly(D,L-lactic acid) nanoparticles by an emulsification-diffusion technique, Int. J. Pharm. 143 (1996) 133-141.

[36] D. Quintanar-Guerrero, A. Ganem-Quintanar, E. Allémann, H. Fessi, E. Doelker, Influence of the stabilizer coating layer on the purification and freeze-drying of poly(D,L-lactic acid) nanoparticles prepared by an emulsion-diffusion technique, J. Microencapsul. 15 (1998) 107-119.

[37] D. Quintanar-Guerrero, E. Allémann, H. Fessi, E. Doelker, Pseudolatex preparation using a novel emulsion-diffusion process involving direct displacement of partially water-miscible solvents by distillation, Int. J. Pharm. 188 (1999) 155-164.

[38] E. Allémann, J. Leroux, R. Gurny, Polymeric nano- and microparticles for the oral delivery of peptides and peptidomimetics, Adv. Drug Deliv. Rev. 34 (1998) 171-189.

[39] M. J. Alonso, Nanomedicines for overcoming biological barriers, Biomed. Pharmacother. 58 (2004) 168-172.

[40] L. Brannon-Peppas, Recent advances on the use of biodegradable microparticles and nanoparticles in controlled drug delivery, Int. J. Pharm. 116 (1995) 1-9.

[41] K. S. Soppimath, T. M. Aminabhavi, A. R. Kulkarni, W. E. Rudzinski, Biodegradable polymeric nanoparticles as drug delivery devices, J. Control. Release 70 (2001) 1-20.

[42] P. A. McCarron, A. D. Woolfson, S. M. Keating, Sustained release of 5-fluorouracil from polymeric nanoparticles, J. Pharm. Pharmacol. 52 (2000) 1451-1459.

[43] G. Fontana, G. Pitarresi, V. Tomarchio, B. Carlisi, P. L. San Biagio, Preparation, characterization and *in vitro* antimicrobial activity of ampicillin-loaded polyethylcyanoacrylate nanoparticles, Biomaterials 19 (1998) 1009-1017.

[44] M. Leroueil-Le Verger, L. Fluckiger, Y. I. Kim, M. Hoffman, P. Maincent, Preparation and characterization of nanoparticles containing an antihypertensive agent, Eur. J. Pharm. Biopharm. 46 (1998) 137-143.

[45] H. Murakami, M. Kobayashi, H. Takeuchi, Y. Kawashima, Preparation of poly(D,L-lactide-*co*-glycolide) nanoparticles by modified spontaneous emulsification solvent diffusion method, Int. J. Pharm. 187 (1999) 143-152.

[46] T. Govender, S. Stolnik, M. C. Garnett, L. Illum, S. S. Davis, PLGA nanoparticles prepared by nanoprecipitation: drug loading and release studies of a water soluble drug, J. Control. Release 57 (1999) 171-185.

[47] J. Matsumoto, Y. Nakada, K. Sakurai, T. Nakamura, Y. Takahashi, Preparation of nanoparticles consisted of poly(D,L-lactide)-poly(ethylene glycol)-poly(D,L-lactide) and their evaluation *in vitro*, Int. J. Pharm. 185 (1999) 93-101.

[48] H. Suh, B. Jeong, R. Rathi, S. W. Kim, Regulation of smooth muscle cell proliferation using paclitaxel-loaded poly(ethylene oxide)-poly(lactide/glycolide) nanospheres, J. Biomed. Mater. Res. 42 (1998) 331-338.

[49] T. Verrecchia, G. Spenlehauer, D. V. Bazile, A. Murry-Brelier, Y. Archimbaud, M. Veillard, Non-stealth (poly(lactic acid/albumin)) and stealth (poly(lactic acid-polyethylene glycol)) nanoparticles as injectable drug carriers, J. Control. Release 36 (1995) 49-61.

[50] Y. H. Cheng, L. Illum, S. S. Davis, A poly(D,L-lactide-*co*-glycolide) microsphere depot system for delivery of haloperidol, J. Control. Release 55 (1998) 203-212.

[51] J. C. Leroux, E. Allémann, F. De Jaeghere, E. Doelker, R. Gurny, Biodegradable nanoparticles -- From sustained release formulations to improved site specific drug delivery, J. Control. Release 39 (1996) 339-350.

[52] M. D. Blanco, M. J. Alonso, Development and characterization of protein-loaded poly(lactide-*co*-glycolide) nanospheres, Eur. J. Pharm. Biopharm. 43 (1997) 287-294.

[53] M. Tobio, A. Sanchez, A. Vila, I. Soriano, C. Evora, J. L. Vila-Jato, M. J. Alonso, The role of PEG on the stability in digestive fluids and *in vivo* fate of PEG-PLA nanoparticles following oral administration, Colloids Surf. B 18 (2000) 315-323.

[54] S. Nicoli, P. Santi, P. Couvreur, G. Couarraze, P. Colombo, E. Fattal, Design of triptorelin loaded nanospheres for transdermal iontophoretic administration, Int. J. Pharm. 214 (2001) 31-35.

CHAPITRE II

PRÉPARATION ET CARACTÉRISATION DE NANOPARTICULES CHARGÉES EN IBUPROFÈNE

Chapitre II

VERSATILITY OF THREE TECHNIQUES FOR PREPARING NANOPARTICLES OF DIFFERENT SIZES AND DRUG LOADINGS

S. Galindo-Rodríguez [1,2,3], *E. Allémann* [2], *E. Doelker* [2] and *H. Fessi* [3]

[1] Pharmapeptides, Geneva-Lyon Interuniversity Center, 74166 Archamps, France.

[2] School of Pharmacy, University of Geneva, 1211 Geneva 4, Switzerland.

[3] UMR-CNRS 5007, Faculty of Pharmacy, Claude Bernard University Lyon I, Lyon, France.

Submitted to Journal of Drug Delivery Science and Technology

Abstract

Comparative studies of the techniques used for preparing polymeric nanoparticles (NP) are rarely reported in the literature. To gain insight in this field, NP were prepared under different conditions using the salting-out, emulsification-diffusion and nanoprecipitation methods and their properties such as drug loading efficiency, residual poly(vinyl alcohol), thermal behavior and morphological characteristics were investigated. Methacrylic acid copolymer Type C (Eudragit® L100-55) and ibuprofen (IBU) were used as polymer and model drug, respectively. The salting-out and emulsification-diffusion methods allowed the preparation of IBU-loaded NP with the mean sizes ranging from 140 to 650 nm. Drug loading efficiency was improved when the NP mean size increased and the aqueous phase pH decreased. Nanoprecipitation allowed production of NP with sub-140 nm mean size. IBU was more effectively incorporated in salting-out-NP than in emulsification-diffusion-NP. Basically, the inherent formulation parameters of the salting-out method — i.e. lower solubility of Eudragit® L100-55 in acetone, miscibility of acetone with water and lower volume of water required to induce solvent diffusion — favored the polymer precipitation rate and solvent diffusion rate, promoting drug incorporation into the NP. Nanoprecipitation resulted in poor IBU incorporation into the NP. Differential scanning calorimetry studies revealed that IBU was present in an amorphous or molecularly dispersed state in the NP.

Keywords: Nanoparticles – Salting-out – Nanoprecipitation – Emulsification-diffusion – Ibuprofen – Eudragit L100-55 – Poly(vinyl alcohol) – Solvent in water diffusion coefficient.

Préparation et caractérisation de nanoparticules chargées en ibuprofène

---

INTRODUCTION

Nanoparticles (NP) have been investigated as drug delivery systems for both oral and parenteral administration routes. They can offer several advantages for the incorporated drug, including protection against degradation, controlled release, prolongation of the circulation time, and targeting to specific sites of action (organ or tissue). In addition, delivery of biological molecules (e.g., proteins, peptides and oligonucleotides) can be also obtained with these colloidal carriers. The characteristics of NP can be modified by several strategies: i) use of natural and synthetic polymers, which change the chemical nature of the polymeric matrix, ii) incorporation of active molecules (e.g. invasins, lectins), which add or inhibit a specific biological property of the carrier, and iii) application of different methods of NP preparation in order to modify their internal and external structures. Importantly, the preparation method can not only modify the physicochemical characteristics of NP such as size, porosity, roughness and morphology, but also properties such as drug loading, release kinetics and targeting of NP.

In general, the methods for manufacturing NP have been studied individually. Most of the studies have been oriented towards an investigation of the process parameters that affect drug entrapment and particle size. However, very few studies exist in which the performances of these techniques are compared. Comparative studies are an important aid for identifying the most appropriate technique for preparing NP with predefined characteristics in terms of size, surface properties, drug loading and drug release. In a previous study, we investigated the main formulation parameters that influenced the formation of NP produced by the salting-out, emulsification-diffusion and nanoprecipitation methods [1]. Therefore, the present study was focused on examining the incorporation of a slightly water soluble drug in NP prepared by these three techniques. Ibuprofen (IBU), Eudragit® L 100-55 (E L100-55) and poly(vinyl alcohol) (PVAL) were used as model drug, polymer and emulsifying agent, respectively. The physicochemical characteristics of the NP were assessed in terms of size, residual PVAL, thermal behaviour and morphology. Special emphasis was placed on interpreting differences of drug loading efficiency.

Ibuprofen was selected as a model drug because of its physicochemical characteristics and pharmacological properties. The salting-out, emulsification-diffusion and nanoprecipitation methods have been successfully used for encapsulation of highly hydrophobic drugs. However, they have shown certain limitations with respect to the encapsulation of hydrophilic compounds. Therefore, being slightly soluble in water and having a pKa = 5.3, IBU was a good candidate to evaluate the ability of incorporation of a slightly water-soluble drug as well as different formulation parameters (i.e., influence of pH on the NP drug loading) of these three techniques. From a pharmaceutical point of view, a dosage form based on IBU-loaded NP could also be of interest. Bucolo et al. [2] observed that , following ocular administration, the local activity of IBU was improved when it was incorporated into NP. Orally administered, IBU-loaded NP might be also helpful. As demonstrated for other anti-inflammatory drugs, the gastrointestinal irritation induced by IBU [3] could be minimized by using particulate systems [4].

I. MATERIALS AND METHODS

1. Materials

Ibuprofen was kindly supplied by Laboratoires UPSA (Rueil-Malmaison, France). Poly(vinyl alcohol), with a molecular weight of 26 000 and a hydrolysis degree of 88% (Mowiol® 4-88, Hoechst), was a gift from Omya AG (Oftringen, Switzerland). Methacrylic acid copolymer Type C NF/USP (Eudragit® L 100-55, Röhm Pharma Polymers) was a gift from Röhm GmbH & Co. KG (Darmstadt, Germany). All other chemicals used were of reagent grade.

2. Methods

2.1. Preparation of nanoparticles

The NP were prepared according to standard procedures of the salting-out [5], emulsification-diffusion [6], and nanoprecipitation [7] methods. In some cases, the general procedures were modified in order to study different aspects of these techniques.

Salting-out. Typically, 50 g of aqueous solution of magnesium chloride hexahydrate (30.4 %, w/w) and PVAL (5.0 to 17.0 %, w/w) were added under mechanical stirring to 30 g of an organic phase containing 9.0 % of E L100-55 and 1.0 % (w/w) of IBU in acetone. Stirring was maintained at 2000 rpm for 15 min. After emulsification, 50 g of pure water were added to induce the diffusion of the organic solvent in water and the formation of NP.

23

Emulsification-diffusion. For this method, 30 g of an aqueous solution of PVAL (7.0 to 17.0 %, w/w) were added under stirring to 21 g of an organic solution of polymer and drug in benzyl alcohol (14.3 and 1.4 %, w/w, respectively). The resulting o/w emulsion was stirred continuously at 2000 rpm for 15 min. Then, 660 g of water were introduced in order to allow the diffusion of the organic solvent into the aqueous external phase, leading to NP formation.

Nanoprecipitation. The polymer (360 mg) and the drug (36 mg) were dissolved in acetone (25 ml). The organic solution was added into the aqueous phase (50 ml) containing PVAL (0.4 %, w/w) and stirred magnetically. The solvent was then evaporated under reduced pressure.

2.2. Nanoparticle purification

Nanoparticles were separated from free surfactant by centrifugation (Centrifuge model Avanti 30 and Ultracentrifuge model LF, both Beckman Instruments, California, U.S.A.). They were washed four times using 30 ml of water adjusted to pH = 3.0 with concentrated HCl and finally with deionised water. After recovery, the washed NP were freeze-dried (LSL Secfroid, model Lyolab BII, Switzerland).

2.3. Determination of particle size

Mean particle size distribution and polydispersity of raw NP were assessed by photon correlation spectroscopy (Zetasizer 3000®, Malvern Instruments, Worcestershire, U.K.) dispersing the NP in deionised water. With respect to the polydispersity index (P.I.), which ranged from 0 to 1, a higher value corresponds to a less homogeneous NP size distribution.

2.4. Drug loading efficiency

An exactly weighed amount of freeze-dried NP was dissolved in 0.1 M NaOH. The samples were assayed for IBU concentration by UV spectroscopy (Hewlett Packard 8453 Spectrophotometer, Germany) at the wavelength of maximum absorbance (λ_{max} = 272 nm). Drug loading efficiency was the ratio between the experimentally measured ibuprofen content and the theoretical value expressed as a percentage.

2.5. Residual poly(vinyl alcohol)

Nanoparticles were assayed for residual PVAL using a method that involves the formation of a stable complex of PVAL with iodine in presence of boric acid [8]. First, freeze-dried NP were dissolved in 0.1 M NaOH. Subsequently, E L100-55 was precipitated by the addition of 0.1 M HCl and the suspension centrifuged. For the PVAL determination, an aliquot of supernatant was treated with 7.5 ml of boric acid solution (4.0 %, w/v) and 1.5 ml of iodine solution (1.27 % iodine and 2.50 % potassium iodide in distilled water, w/v), adjusting the volume to 25.0 ml with water. Finally, the absorbance was measured at 644 nm.

2.6. Scanning electron microscopy

Morphological examination of NP was performed using a scanning electron microscope (model JEOL JSM-6400, Jeol Ltd., Japan). Samples of dried NP were dispersed in water. Subsequently, drops of suspension were dried in air over metallic studs and coated with gold.

2.7. Differential scanning calorimetry

Thermal analysis was carried out on samples of E L100-55, IBU, PVAL and NP using a differential scanning calorimeter (model DSC 220 C, Seiko Instruments, Inc). The samples were performed at a scanning rate of 10 $^{\circ}$C min^{-1}, from 20 to 200 $^{\circ}$C.

II. RESULTS AND DISCUSSION

In order to evaluate the advantages and limitations associated only to the preparation procedure of each method, the study was carried out using the same raw materials (drug, polymer and surfactant) for the three techniques. Discussion of results is mainly focused on analysis of the physicochemical factors influencing drug loading efficiency of NP. Analysis was first oriented to differences between the emulsion-based methods (salting-out and emulsification-diffusion); subsequently, comparison was made with data from the nanoprecipitation method.

1. Effect of pH of the aqueous phase and purification medium on drug loading efficiency

Depending on the pH, the degree of ionization of IBU changes and hence its aqueous solubility [9]. In practice, IBU can migrate either from the emulsion droplets into the external aqueous phase during the emulsification and diffusion steps of NP preparation, or from the NP into the purification media during the washing step of NP purification. Therefore, in order to establish the optimal aqueous conditions to minimize IBU partition, experiments were carried out adjusting the pH in the aqueous phase as well as in the purification medium.

Table I shows the influence of an acidic pH adjustment on drug loading efficiency.

For the salting-out method, adjusting the pH of the aqueous phase and purification medium resulted in a higher drug loading efficiency (79 % for batch SA-B) than in the absence of pH adjustment (66 % for batch SA-A). The same trend was observed in the emulsification-diffusion method (batches ED-B and ED-A, respectively). Basically, in both techniques, lowering pH decreased IBU water solubility and reduced IBU migration into the aqueous phase and the purification medium which enhanced IBU incorporation into the NP.

The number of washing cycles used during NP purification was also considered. It was only studied for the emulsification-diffusion method. As mentioned earlier, purification by centrifugation was carried out in order to eliminate free surfactant from the raw dispersion of NP. However, the number of cycles is very important because during NP purification IBU could also be eliminated from the NP. Batches ED-B and ED-C (*Table I*) were prepared and purified using the same conditions. Only the number of purification cycles was modified, being 3 for ED-B and 5 for ED-C. As can be seen in *Table I*, there is no difference between the drug loading efficiencies of these batches (60 and 59 %, respectively). This is of interest because, for eliminating more PVAL from NP surface, it is possible to increase the number of purification cycles without affecting the drug loading efficiency.

Table I - Effect of the aqueous medium pH on the drug loading efficiency of nanoparticles prepared by salting-out, emulsification–diffusion and nanoprecipitation (Mean ± SD, n=3)

Method and batch	Mean size (nm) and polydispersity index [P.I.] [a]	Aqueous phase pH	Purification medium pH [b]	Drug loading efficiency (%) [c]
Salting-out				
SA-A	295 ± 5 [0.11 ± 0.07]	Not-adjusted	Not-adjusted	66 ± 3
SA-B	281 ± 7 [0.09 ± 0.05]	1.5	3.0	79 ± 4
Emulsification-diffusion				
ED-A	282 ± 10 [0.11 ± 0.04]	Not-adjusted	Not-adjusted	51 ± 2
ED-B	279 ± 9 [0.08 ± 0.05]	1.5	3.0*	60 ± 3
ED-C	292 ± 5 [0.12 ± 0.03]	1.5	3.0	59 ± 2
Nanoprecipitation				
NPR-A	141 ± 3 [0.15 ± 0.07]	Not-adjusted	Not-adjusted	38 ± 3
NPR-B	Poor NP formation [d]	1.5	3.0	------- [d]
NPR-C	137 ± 3 [0.14 ± 0.06]	Not-adjusted	3.0	39 ± 2

[a, c] Mean size and drug loading efficiency result of three determinations from three different batches. For P.I., which ranges from 0 to 1, a higher value indicates a less homogeneous NP size distribution.

[b] In all cases purification was performed employing five washing cycles, except for batch marked with (*) for which three cycle s were used.

[d] Drug loading efficiency was not determined because NP recovery was highly affected. Approximately, 65 % of polymer precipitated as amorphous aggregates.

28

The effect of pH adjustment was also assessed for the nanoprecipitation method. A first batch (NPR-A) was prepared without pH adjustment resulting in NP with a mean size of 141 nm [0.15] and a drug loading efficiency of 38 %. The second batch (NPR-B) was produced by adjusting the aqueous phase to pH = 1.5. In this case, the results were deceptive because, even though NP were obtained, part of the polymer precipitated forming amorphous aggregates which dramatically affected NP yield. The aggregates corresponded to 65 % of initial polymer weight. Although similar results have been reported when preparing NP by nanoprecipitation, this behavior cannot be generalized because in other studies pH adjustment of the aqueous phase gave satisfactory results [10].The differences are probably due to the type of polymer and its aggregation behavior which is influenced by the ionic strength in the aqueous phase. It may be also conceivable that pH change has some influence on polymer precipitation kinetics. Nevertheless, pH adjustment could be considered disadvantageous for the nanoprecipitation method because, in order to increase the drug loading of ionizable drugs, this might not give favorable results. Finally, in a third batch (NPR-C), NP were prepared by adjusting the pH of the purification medium (pH = 3.0), but not that of the aqueous phase. Compared to NPR-A, its particle mean size was relatively similar (137 nm [0.14]) but the drug loading efficiency (39 %) was not improved. This means that changing pH in the purification medium does not have an influence on the drug loading of NP prepared by nanoprecipitation.

As a consequence, for the next steps of this study, the batches prepared by salting-out and emulsification-diffusion were produced using an aqueous phase adjusted to pH = 1.5 and a purification medium at pH = 3.0. For NP purification, five washing cycles were performed. In the case of the nanoprecipitation method, aqueous phase and purification medium were used without pH adjustment.

2. Drug loading efficiency by the emulsion-based methods

Since the results will be analyzed in terms of the mechanism of NP formation, a brief description of the physicochemical phenomena involved will now be given. In the emulsion-based techniques, such as salting-out and emulsification-diffusion, a nanoemulsion is first formed during NP preparation [1]. In this primary emulsion the droplets are constituted by the polymer, drug and solvent. Subsequently, during the dilution-diffusion step, a sufficient amount of water is added to the emulsion in order to extract the solvent from the droplets and induce NP formation. In fact, drug entrapment occurs when the polymer chains desolvate forming a dense solid network which immobilizes the drug. Both phenomena, solvent diffusion and polymer precipitation, occur simultaneously and they are intimately related to drug loading because during these processes a part of the drug can also diffuse with the solvent into the external aqueous phase. From a practical point of view, a rapid polymer desolvation is preferable in order to limit the drug leakage during the solvent diffusion and favor drug loading [11,12].

2.1. Influence of nanoparticle mean size on the drug loading efficiency

For salting-out and emulsification-diffusion, NP with different mean particle sizes were obtained by stirring at 2000 rpm and varying the emulsifier concentration in the external phase (*Table II*).

Table II - Mean particle size and polydispersity index [P.I.] of nanoparticles prepared by salting-out, emulsification-diffusion and nanoprecipitation (Mean ± SD, n=3)

Nominal diameter (nm)	Mean particle size (nm) and P.I. [a]		
	Salting-out	Emulsification-diffusion	Nanoprecipitation
650	653 ± 35 [0.57 ± 0.14]	671 ± 57 [0.52 ± 0.16]	
450	441 ± 72 [0.52 ± 0.21]	455 ± 32 [0.43 ± 0.19]	
300	287 ± 9 [0.11 ± 0.03]	292 ± 5 [0.11 ± 0.04]	
140	141 ± 5 [0.04 ± 0.02]	141 ± 3 [0.07 ± 0.02]	147 ± 7 [0.09 ± 0.02]

[a] Polydispersity index ranges from 0 to 1. A higher value indicates a less homogeneous NP size distribution.

Table III - Ibuprofen-loading efficiency [a] and residual PVAL [a] of nanoparticles prepared by the salting-out, emulsification-diffusion and nanoprecipitation methods

Diameter (nm)	Salting-out		Emulsification-diffusion		Nanoprecipitation	
	Loading efficiency (%)	Residual PVAL (%)	Loading efficiency (%)	Residual PVAL (%)	Loading efficiency (%)	Residual PVAL (%)
650	93	2.8	70	3.7		
450	85	3.1	64	5.2		
300	79	4.9	60	5.3		
140	68	12.9	55	10.9	42	3.5

[a] Drug loading efficiency and residual PVAL data were obtained from three determinations from three different batches.

In the analysis of the results, the NP batches are referred according to their nominal diameter. The effect of particle size on the drug loading efficiency is shown in *Table III*. It can be noted that a decrease in the NP mean size results in a diminution of IBU loading efficiency of NP. In the salting-out-method, drug loading efficiency values varied from 68 to 93 % for NP with mean sizes between 140 and 650 nm, while for the emulsification-diffusion method, the drug loading efficiency ranged from 55 to 70 % for the same interval of mean particle sizes. Considering the mechanism of NP formation, the results can be analyzed regarding the diffusional surface area of nanodroplets with different particle mean size. During the dilution-diffusion step, when water is added to the emulsion, both solvent diffusion and polymer desolvation occur simultaneously from the droplet surface to its internal structure. As mentioned above, part of the drug present in the droplets also diffuses with the solvent into the external phase. This mainly occurs during the earlier stage of solvent diffusion because the drug found close to the organic solvent/water droplet interface can be removed more easily than that present in the droplet interior. This is also supported by the fact that a dense film-like wall is formed around the droplet which limits drug diffusion from the internal droplet structure [12,13]. Therefore, assuming first that drug loss during the solvent extraction mainly comes from the surface of the nanodroplets, and second, that a larger diffusional surface is associated with smaller droplets, IBU leakage was more pronounced in smaller NP than in larger ones which yielded lower drug loading efficiency in the smaller NP.

2.2. Drug loading efficiency comparison of nanoparticles prepared by salting-out and emulsification-diffusion

Owing to the differences between the salting-out and emulsification-diffusion techniques, basically in the physicochemical characteristics of their organic and aqueous phases and in the solvent-diffusion process, it was also expected that there would be differences in the drug loading efficiencies of NP produced by each method. Comparing at the same nominal particle size, in all cases IBU was more effectively encapsulated in NP prepared by salting-out than those for emulsification-diffusion (*Table III*). For instance, 300 nm-NP have IBU contents of 60 and 79 %, for NP prepared by emulsification-diffusion and salting-out, respectively. The polymer solubility in the organic phase and the water-solubility of the organic solvent, both of them associated to polymer precipitation rate, were the factors considered to explain these results.

An important property of the polymers is their solubility in organic solvents. The solubility determines the rate of hardening (solidification) of the polymer chains during NP preparation. The solubility of E L100-55, which is evidenced by the physical appearance of the organic solution, is markedly different in acetone and in benzyl alcohol. A transparent system was obtained when E L100-55 was dissolved in benzyl alcohol which indicates that the solvent acts as a "good solvent" for the polymer. In contrast, a turbid system resulted when acetone was used as a solvent which means that the solvent interacts as a "poor solvent" with the polymer. This is an important difference because a particular behaviour reflects the extent of polymer-polymer and polymer-solvent interactions. In a "good solvent" polymer chains are more disentangled from one another, and hence are extensively solvated. Conversely, in a "poor solvent" chains of polymer are more shrunken and their solvation is limited. In other words, whilst polymer-solvent interaction is favored in a "good solvent", polymer-polymer interaction is more pronounced in a "poor solvent". As a consequence, the close interaction among the polymers chains in a "poor solvent" make them precipitate more rapidly when the solvent diffuses into the external aqueous phase. As acetone acts as a "poor solvent" for E L100-55, the polymer chains of E L100-55 precipitate more rapidly and this could prevent IBU diffusion into the external phase promoting a higher drug loading efficiency in the NP prepared by salting-out.

The water-solubility of the organic solvent is another important factor related to drug loading, mainly because it is associated with solvent diffusion rate into the aqueous phase, and then to polymer precipitation rate [11,14]. At the early stage of solvent diffusion, it has been proposed that solvent diffuses from the surface of the droplet and induces polymer hardening forming a dense viscous interface wall [13,15,16]. Adding more water, polymer hardening gradually moves towards the center, immobilizing the drug and preventing its loss into the external phase. This means that polymer precipitation, closely related to the solvent diffusion rate, should take place as early as possible in order to preserve the drug content during the solvent diffusion. Therefore, because diffusion rate of an organic solvent depends on its water solubility, the analysis is done correlating both properties and relating them to the polymer precipitation rate. Solvents with very low water solubility, like benzyl alcohol (*Table IV*), diffuse very slowly into the aqueous continuous phase. In this case, the droplets of the emulsion remain in the liquid state for a long time, and then IBU can easily diffuse across the non-precipitated structure of the droplet. This results in a significant loss of drug to the aqueous phase prior to precipitation. In contrast, being miscible in water, acetone rapidly diffuses and instantaneously precipitates the E L100-55; thus, avoiding simultaneous IBU diffusion. Although, this first empirical approach is convenient for explaining differences in drug loading efficiency of NP prepared by salting-out and emulsification-diffusion, this phenomenon can be more clearly elucidated by considering the ratio of the diffusion coefficient of solvent in water ($D^o_{\text{solvent-water}}$) to that of water in solvent ($D^o_{\text{water-solvent}}$) for both organic solvents. The diffusion coefficients were estimated from the equation proposed by Tyn and Calus [17]:

$$D^o_{solvent_1-solvent_2} = 8.93 \, x \, 10^{-8} \left(\frac{V_{solvent_1}}{V^2_{solvent_2}} \right)^{1/6} \left(\frac{P_{solvent_2}}{P_{solvent_1}} \right)^{3/5} \frac{T}{\eta_{solvent_2}} \qquad \text{Eq. 1}$$

where V is the molar volume at normal boiling temperature, T is the temperature and η is the viscosity. The parachor parameters, P_{solvent} and P_{water}, were obtained from additive group contribution [18]. Calculated diffusion coefficient ratios for benzyl alcohol and acetone (*Table IV*) were of 2.32 and 0.24, respectively. This diffusivity ranking confirms the relationship between the solvent diffusion rate and drug loading efficiency in NP.

Table IV - Related physicochemical properties of acetone and benzyl alcohol

Solvent	Solubility in water (v:v)	Diffusion coefficient [a] ($\times 10^5$ cm^2 s^{-1})		$R = \dfrac{D^0_{solvent-water}}{D^0_{water-solvent}}$
		D^o solvent-water	D^o water-solvent	
Acetone	miscible	1.34	5.61	0.24
Benzyl alcohol	1:60	0.95	0.41	2.32

[a] Calculated from *Equation 1*.

Compared with benzyl alcohol used in emulsification-diffusion, acetone was extracted more rapidly from the emulsion droplet and promoted a rapid polymer precipitation at the droplet interface which, in turn, limited drug migration into the aqueous phase. As a result, drug loading efficiency was higher in NP prepared by salting-out than in those prepared by emulsification-diffusion.

2.2.1. Influence of dilution water volume on the drug loading. As mentioned earlier, drug can migrate into the external phase during the dilution-diffusion step. Basically, adding water for solvent diffusion increases the number of water molecules that can interact, and thus dissolve the drug located at the vicinity of the droplet surface. So, the volume of water used for the dilution-diffusion step of each technique is also considered to explain the differences in drug loading efficiencies of salting-out-NP and emulsification-diffusion-NP. The marked difference in the dilution water volume employed in each method is shown by the dilution ratio (ratio$_{dil}$ = volume of water used for dilution/volume of dispersed phase) which relates the volume of dilution-water by volume unit of internal phase. The dilution ratios for salting-out (ratio$_{dil, SA}$) and emulsification-diffusion (ratio$_{dil, ED}$) correspond to 1.7 and 31.4, respectively. Considering the difference between these values, it can be appreciated that a volume of internal phase used in emulsification-diffusion might potentially interact some 20-fold more with the water present than a volume of internal phase used in salting-out. This suggests that IBU diffusion from the internal phase might be substantially more pronounced in the emulsification-diffusion technique than in salting-out. Therefore, a larger volume of water added during the dilution-diffusion step, which provided a larger dispersion area, increases the water-IBU interaction leading to the extraction of more drug molecules from the droplet. It also contributes to the higher drug loading efficiencies of NP prepared by salting-out.

2.2.2. Presence of salts in the external phase. Another formulation variable to be considered is the high concentration of $MgCl_2$ in the external phase of the salting-out method which can influence drug loading. In fact, the use of salts in the continuous aqueous phase has been often tested to improve the encapsulation of drug in particulate systems prepared by emulsion-based methods [19,20]. Since the presence of $MgCl_2$ (30.4 %, w/w) in the aqueous phase used in salting-out diminishes IBU water solubility, IBU diffusion into the external phase during emulsification and diffusion steps is limited. As a result, this contributes to enhancing the drug loading efficiency in NP prepared by salting-out compared to those made by emulsification-diffusion.

2.3. Residual poly(vinyl alcohol) in nanoparticles prepared by salting-out, emulsification-diffusion and nanoprecipitation

For the salting-out and emulsification-diffusion methods, PVAL content in the aqueous phase was varied in order to obtain NP with different mean sizes. Increasing the PVAL concentration in the external phase allows NP of mean sizes from 650 to 140 nm to be obtained. The role of PVAL as an emulsifier is manifold and has been extensively discussed in previous work [1]. Briefly, during the emulsification step, PVAL decreases the droplet size and then the NP mean size through different stabilization mechanisms. Whilst interacting in the bulk solution, PVAL promotes hydrodynamic stabilization; its presence at the emulsion droplet interface enables PVAL to reduce the interfacial tension as well as to induce the steric and mechanical stabilizations. In particular, as a consequence of its interaction at the droplet interface, PVAL remains at the particle surface even after intensive and repeated washing cycles. The binding of PVAL on the NP surface is likely to happen when the organic solvent is removed from the interface in which interpenetration of PVAL and E L100-55 chains takes place [1].

2.3.1. Relationship between mean size of nanoparticles and residual poly(vinyl alcohol)

In the present study, residual PVAL was assayed in NP of different mean sizes. Nanoparticles were previously purified by centrifugation employing five washing cycles and freeze dried. As is illustrated in *Table III*, a decrease in the NP mean size is associated with an increase in the residual PVAL. The NP mean sizes of 650 to 140 nm correspond to values of residual PVAL between 2.8–12.9 % for salting-out and 3.7–10.9 % for emulsification-diffusion, respectively. This can be related to the increase in surface area of NP. During emulsification, decreasing the size of nanodroplets results in an extensive increase of the exposed surface of the internal phase which is covered and stabilized by PVAL chains. Following solvent diffusion, PVAL chains remain on the NP surface resulting in higher values of residual PVAL. Therefore, the smaller the mean size, the larger surface area, and the more PVAL molecules adsorbed at the NP surface.

2.3.2. Effect of preparation method on the residual poly(vinyl alcohol)

Comparison of NP with the same mean size, in all cases shows that NP prepared by salting-out have lower residual PVAL values than those produced by emulsification-diffusion. For instance, at a nominal mean size of 450 nm, NP prepared by salting-out and emulsification-diffusion exhibit residual PVAL percentages of 3.1 and 5.2, respectively. These results can be explained from the interpenetration phenomenon [1]. Since interpenetration is due to mutual diffusion of PVAL and E L100-55 chains through the droplet interface, the E

L100-55 conformation in the organic solvent plays an important role in formation of the interpenetrated network. Acetone was used as solvent in the organic phase of the salting-out method whereas benzyl alcohol was the solvent in emulsification-diffusion. As mentioned earlier, they act as "poor solvent" and "good solvent" for E L100-55, respectively. It means that chains of E L100-55 are unfolded and more extended in benzyl alcohol than in acetone. This conformation, in which polymer chains are more solvated, allows E L100-55 chains to diffuse more easily into the interface and to interact more intimately with the present PVAL chains. In contrast, the shrunken chains of E L100-55 in acetone reduce their surface area hindering the PVAL–E L100-55 interactions at the interface. Therefore, because interpenetration of PVAL–E L100-55 is better achieved when benzyl alcohol is used like a solvent, more PVAL molecules can remain at the NP surface, and thereby a higher percentage of residual PVAL is obtained in NP prepared by emulsification-diffusion than those by salting-out.

In contrast to the emulsion-based methods, the emulsifying agent concentration does not influence the mean size of NP prepared by nanoprecipitation. In fact, NP can be obtained in the absence of surfactant. It is only necessary for NP that need to be maintained in suspension for a long time. Because PVAL concentration in the aqueous phase was not varied, residual PVAL was only assessed for 140 nm-NP. In this case, a direct comparison with the NP prepared by salting-out and emulsification-diffusion is not feasible because NP formation is independent of PVAL concentration in the aqueous phase. However, it is remarkable that when PVAL is present in the aqueous phase, it remains on the NP even after purification. It means that NP prepared by nanoprecipitation can be obtained with or without PVAL. This is particularly important because absence or presence of residual PVAL at the surface of NP can change their physicochemical and biological behavior. The choice of one or another type of NP will depend on the requirements of NP preparation which obviously represents an advantage from the stand point of formulation. Furthermore, it is of interest to mention that surfactant-free NP cannot be produced by the salting-out and emulsification-diffusion methods. However, it should be noted that the PVAL layer on the NP does present some interesting features as it promotes an almost-instantaneous redispersion of the freeze-dried particles in water, it improves the stability of NP suspensions against flocculation in water, it allows adsorption of other substrates leading to change NP surface characteristics, and it modifies NP biorecognition.

2.4. Differential scanning calorimetry

In order to evaluate whether the IBU loaded in NP was in an amorphous or a crystalline state, differential scanning calorimetry (DSC) analysis was carried out on samples of individual substances as well as NP free of IBU and IBU-loaded NP. The DSC profile for pure IBU (*Figure 1-A*) shows an endothermic peak of melting at 73.7 °C and an enthalpy of fusion (ΔH_f) of 144.16 mJ/mg. The sharpness of the peak indicates that IBU was in a crystalline form. The thermal analysis of NP prepared by salting-out and emulsification-diffusion are shown in *Figures 1-B and 1-C*, respectively.

In both cases, the thermograms of the NP free of IBU show only one endothermic event which occurs approximately between 65 and 120 °C. Regarding the DSC curves of IBU-loaded NP, in addition to the above thermal transition, an endothermic peak can be observed at ~60 °C which corresponds to a shifted melting transition of IBU. These peaks were significantly broader and

41

showed a lower onset with respect to the endothermic peak of the pure IBU. In particular, for IBU-loaded NP prepared by salting-out, the endothermic peak showed a ΔH_f = 1.25 mJ/mg. Considering that IBU-loading of NP was 6.3 %, this ΔH_f corresponded to 3.0 % of the ΔH_f for the pure crystalline drug. In the case of IBU-loaded NP prepared by emulsification-diffusion and containing 6.2 % of drug, the resulting ΔH_f = 1.30 mJ/mg corresponded to 2.7 % of the ΔH_f of the crystalline pure drug.

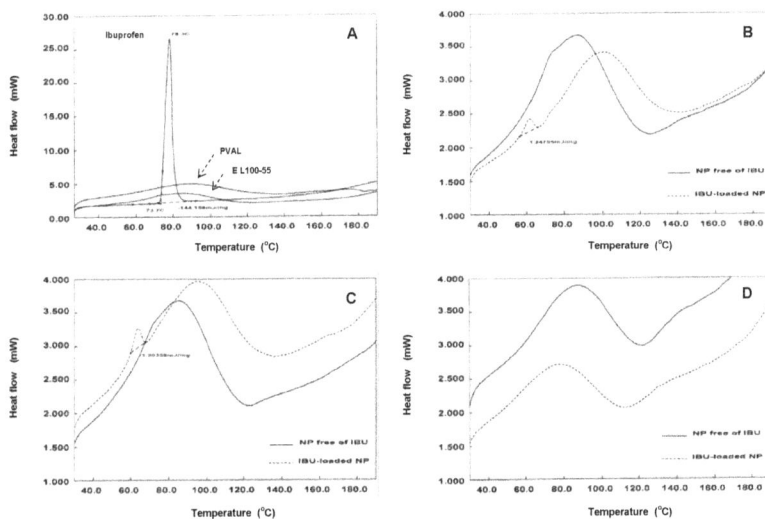

Figure 1 - DSC thermograms obtained for IBU, PVAL and E L100-55 (A) as well as for nanoparticles prepared by the salting-out (B), emulsification-diffusion (C) and nanoprecipitation (D) methods.

These results suggest that most of the drug is incorporated in an amorphous state or is molecularly dispersed in the polymer matrix. In NP prepared by nanoprecipitation, having a drug loading of 3.4 %, this phenomenon was more evident. Clearly, no endothermic transition corresponding to the IBU fusion was observed in the curve of IBU-loaded NP (*Figure 1-D*). As reported by other authors [21], the absence or low crystallinity of IBU, when it was incorporated in particulate systems, is attributed to the low drug content of the NP. Basically, because the drug molecules are found relatively diluted in the polymer matrix, its nucleation to form crystalline structures is prevented, and thus they tend to precipitate forming a molecular dispersion with the polymer.

2.5. Scanning electron microscopy

Figure 2 shows representative scanning electron micrographs of IBU-loaded NP obtained from the three methods.

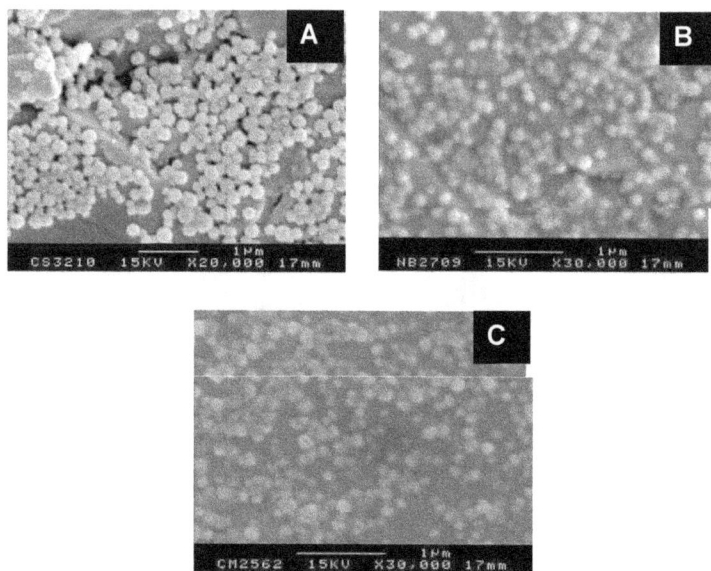

Figure 2 - Scanning electron microphotographs of ibuprofen-loaded nanoparticles prepared by emulsification-diffusion (A), salting-out (B) and nanoprecipitation (C).

The NP produced by emulsification-diffusion (*Figure 2-A*) had a spherical shape as well as a homogeneous particle size distribution (180-260 nm). For salting-out, scanning electron micrographs (*Figure 2-B*) revealed fine spherical NP of sub-160 nm diameter also possessing great homogeneity. Finally, relatively monodispersed particles with well defined spherical shape are observed for NP prepared by nanoprecipitation (*Figure 2-C*). Most of the particles are in the size range 100-140 nm. In all cases, it can be confirmed that there is neither aggregation nor adhesion among the NP.

III. CONCLUSIONS

The IBU-loaded NP were successfully prepared by the salting-out, emulsification-diffusion and nanoprecipitation methods. The effect of the process variables of these techniques on the physicochemical characteristics of the resulting NP was also investigated. A mechanistic approach, which involved the physicochemical phenomena associated with NP formation, was proposed to explain differences of drug loading efficiency, residual PVAL and the thermal behavior of NP.

In the salting-out and emulsification-diffusion methods, decreasing the aqueous external medium pH to 1.5 reduced the aqueous IBU solubility thereby enhancing the drug loading efficiency of NP. Moreover, broad ranges of mean NP sizes, from 140 to 650 nm, were obtained by both methods and a close relationship between drug loading efficiency and NP mean size was also observed. Significantly more IBU was incorporated in larger NP than in smaller ones. This behavior is attributed to the larger diffusional surface area of smaller precursor nanodroplets which facilitate the IBU leakage into the external aqueous phase during dilution-diffusion step. Comparing NP of the same size,

NP prepared by salting-out presented higher drug loading efficiencies than those produced by emulsification-diffusion. Basically, lower solubility of E L100-55 in acetone, miscibility of acetone in water and lower volume of water used in the solvent-diffusion step of the salting-out method were all factors promoting polymer precipitation rate and solvent-diffusion rate, which in turn enhanced the IBU incorporation into the NP. For the nanoprecipitation method, only sub-140 nm IBU-loaded NP were prepared. In addition, pH adjustment of the aqueous phase was not possible for this technique because large amorphous polymer aggregates were formed in addition to the NP affecting significantly NP yield. The scanning electron micrographs revealed that NP with a well defined spherical shape and great homogeneity can be obtained by the three preparation methods of NP. Furthermore, DSC studies suggest that the IBU associated to NP was molecularly dispersed within the polymeric network. In conclusion, it can be stated that it is possible to prepare a wide variety of IBU-loaded NP in terms of size and drug loading efficiency by the three methods which would offer numerous possibilities for the modulation of certain pharmaceutical and biological properties of NP including, drug release, bioadhesion, oral uptake and targeting.

ACKNOWLEDGEMENTS

S. Galindo-Rodriguez was supported by a grant from CONACYT-SFERE (México-France). He also acknowledges FES-Cuautitlán, UNAM, México. The authors are grateful to Mrs C. Siegfried and N. Boulens for their technical assistance in the SEM and Dr. Y. Kalia for critically reviewing the manuscript.

Chapitre II

References

1 GALINDO-RODRIGUEZ S., ALLEMANN E., FESSI H., DOELKER E. - Physicochemical parameters associated with nanoparticle formation in the salting-out, emulsification-diffusion, and nanoprecipitation methods. - Pharm. Res., **21**, 1428-1439, 2004.

2 BUCOLO C., MALTESE A., PUGLISI G., PIGNATELLO R. - Enhanced ocular anti-inflammatory activity of ibuprofen carried by an Eudragit^R RS100 nanoparticle suspension. – Ophthalmic Res., **34**, 319-323, 2002.

3 CIOLI V., PUTZOLU S., ROSSI V., SCORZA BARCELLONA P., CORRADINO C. - The role of direct tissue contact in the production of gastrointestinal ulcers by anti-inflammatory drugs in rats. - Toxicol. Appl. Pharmacol., **50**, 283-289, 1979.

4 GUTERRES S.S., FESSI H., BARRATT G., PUISIEUX F., DEVISSAGUET J.P. - Poly(D,L-lactide) nanocapsules containing non-steroidal anti- inflammatory drugs: gastrointestinal tolerance following intravenous and oral administration. - Pharm. Res., **12**, 1545-1547, 1995.

5 BINDSCHAEDLER C., GURNY R., DOELKER E. - Process for preparing a powder of water-insoluble polymer which can be redispersed in a liquid phase, the resulting powder and utilization thereof. - Patent WO 88/08011, 1988.

6 LEROUX J.C., ALLEMANN E., DOELKER E., GURNY R. - New approach for the preparation of nanoparticles by an emulsification-diffusion method. - Eur. J. Pharm. Biopharm., **41**, 14-18, 1995.

7 FESSI H., PUISIEUX F., DEVISSAGUET J.P., AMMOURY N., BENITA S. - Nanocapsule formation by interfacial polymer deposition following solvent displacement. - Int. J. Pharm., **55**, R1-R4, 1989.

8 FINLEY J.H., Spectrophotometric determination of polyvinyl alcohol in paper coatings. - Anal. Chem., **33**, 1925-1927, 1961.

9 HERZFELDT C.D., KUMMEL R. - Dissociation constants, solubilities and dissolution rates of some selected nonsteroidal antiinflammatoires. - Drug Dev. Ind. Pharm., **9**, 767-793, 1983.

10 GOVENDER T., STOLNIK S., GARNETT M.C., ILLUM L., DAVIS S.S. - PLGA nanoparticles prepared by nanoprecipitation: drug loading and release studies of a water soluble drug. - J. Control. Release, **57**, 171-185, 1999.

11 MEHTA R.C., THANOO B.C., DELUCA P.P. - Peptide containing microspheres from low molecular weight and hydrophilic poly(d,l-lactide-co-glycolide). - J. Control. Release, **41**, 249-257, 1996.

12 BODMEIER R., MCGINITY J.W. - Solvent selection in the preparation of poly(DL-lactide) microspheres prepared by the solvent evaporation method. - Int. J. Pharm., **43**, 179-186, 1988.

13 CROTTS G., PARK T.G. - Preparation of porous and nonporous biodegradable polymeric hollow microspheres. - J. Control. Release, **35**, 91-105, 1995.

14 BODMEIER R., CHEN H. - Preparation and characterization of microspheres containing the anti-inflammatory agents, indomethacin, ibuprofen, and ketoprofen. - J. Control. Release, **10**, 167-175, 1989.

15 WEN I., ANDERSON K.W., MEHTA R.C., DELUCA P.P. - Prediction of solvent removal profile and effect on properties for peptide-loaded PLGA microspheres prepared by solvent extraction/evaporation method. - J. Control. Release, **37**, 199-214, 1995.

16 JEYANTHI R., THANOO B.C., METHA R.C., DELUCA P.P. - Effect of solvent removal technique on the matrix characteristics of polylactide/glycolide microspheres for peptide delivery. - J. Control. Release, **38**, 235-244, 1996.

17 Reid C.R., Prausnitz M.J., Poling B.E. - Diffusion coefficients. - In: The Properties of Gases and Liquids, 4th ed., McGraw-Hill, New York, U.S.A., 1986, pp. 577-631.

18 Van Krevelen D.W. - Limiting viscosity number (intrinsic viscosity) and related properties of very diluted solutions. – In: Properties of Polymers, 3rd ed., Elsevier, Amsterdam, Netherlands, 1990, pp. 243-283.

19 KISHIDA A., DRESSMAN J.B., YOSHIOKA S., ASO Y., TAKEDA Y. - Some determinants of morphology and release rate from poly(L)lactic acid microspheres. - J. Control. Release, **13**, 83-89, 1990.

20 AL MAAIEH A., FLANAGAN D.R. - Salt and cosolvent effects on ionic drug loading into microspheres using an O/W method. - J. Control. Release, **70**, 169-181, 2001.

21 DUBERNET C., ROULAND J.C., BENOIT J.P. - Ibuprofen-loaded ethylcellulose microspheres: analysis of the matrix structure by thermal analysis. - J. Pharm. Sci., **80**, 1029-1033, 1991.

CHAPITRE III

TRANSPOSITION D'ÉCHELLE DE TROIS TECHNIQUES DESTINÉES À LA PRÉPARATION DE NANOPARTICULES À BASE DE POLYMÈRES

COMPARATIVE SCALE-UP OF THREE METHODS FOR PRODUCING IBUPROFEN-LOADED NANOPARTICLES

S. Galindo-Rodríguez [1,2,3], *F. Puel* [3], *S. Briançon* [3], *E. Allémann* [2,4], *E. Doelker* [2] *and H. Fessi* [3]

[1] Pharmapeptides, Centre Interuniversitaire de Recherche et d'Enseignement, 74166 Archamps, France.

[2] School of Pharmacy, University of Geneva, 1211 Geneva 4, Switzerland.

[3] Laboratoire d'Automatique et de Génie des Procédés, UMR-CNRS 5007, Université Claude Bernard Lyon I, ESCPE-Lyon Bat. 308G, 43 Bd. du 11 Novembre 1918, 69622 Villeurbanne cedex, France.

[4] Bracco Research SA, Plan-les-Ouates, 1228 Geneva, Switzerland.

Submitted to European Journal of Pharmaceutical Sciences

Abstract

The lack of information related to the scaling-up of technologies used for preparing polymeric nanoparticles (NP) might hinder the introduction of these colloidal carriers into the pharmaceutical market. In the present study, the scale-up of ibuprofen-loaded NP produced by three manufacturing processes – salting-out, emulsification-diffusion and nanoprecipitation – was assessed at pilot-scale by increasing 20-fold the laboratory-batch volume from 60 ml to 1.5 liter. Eudragit® L100-55 and poly(vinyl alcohol) (PVAL) were used as polymer and emulsifying agent, respectively. The influence of the hydrodynamic conditions on the NP characteristics such as mean size, drug content and morphology was also investigated. At pilot-scale, stirring rates of 790 to 2000 rpm lead to NP mean sizes ranging from 557 to 174 nm for salting-out and from 562 to 230 nm for emulsification-diffusion. An increase in the stirring rate enhances the droplet break-up phenomenon which leads to the formation of finer emulsion droplets and thus smaller NP. Moreover, the influence of the stirring rate on the mean size of NP can be predicted using a model based on a simple power law. The continuous

49

method used for nanoprecipitation scale-up allows production of NP in a reproducible way over a relatively short time. Finally, for the three methods, NP characteristics were reproduced well at both scales. However, the scale-up process induced a slight reduction in the size and drug loading of NP.

Keywords: Nanoparticles; Salting-out; Emulsification-diffusion; Nanoprecipitation; Scale-up; Ibuprofen; Drug loading;

1. Introduction

The introduction of a new product on the market is preceded by different stages of research and development. During the course of its development a series of progressive refinements in the formulation, manufacturing processes and product presentation take place. The scale-up phase includes the integration of procedures, as well as the transfer of technology, for realizing the large scale manufacture of a given product. This stage of development is crucial because, very often, many of the process limitations that are not apparent on the small scale become significant on a larger scale, and may even lead to the failure of translating a unit to industrial dimensions. In practice, the transition from a laboratory system to a plant system is not direct. The product is commonly prepared on intermediate scales, larger than the initial development studies but smaller than the industrial manufacturing. Basically, the idea is to simulate production as much as possible and to optimize the operating parameters before large-volume work is performed. A scale-up procedure based on a well prepared technical transfer will assure product quality, overall economy and timely achievement of market readiness.

Although polymeric nanoparticles (NP) have been recognized as one of the most promising colloidal drug delivery systems, their introduction into the pharmaceutical market is likely to be hindered because of a lack of information concerning the scale-up of technologies used for their preparation. The existing information related to this topic is restricted to very few studies (Colombo et al., 2001; Galan Valdivia, et al., 1998; De Labouret et al., 1995). Obviously, with such limited information, efficient scale-up and successful operation at industrial scale is almost impossible. Therefore, in the present study, the scale-up of three manufacturing processes of NP – salting-out, emulsification-diffusion and nanoprecipitation – was assessed by increasing 20-fold the volume of the laboratory batches. The influence of the scale-up, particularly the hydrodynamic parameters, on the NP characteristics such as mean size, drug loading, residual surfactant, and morphology was also investigated. Eudragit$^®$ L100-55, poly(vinyl alcohol) (PVAL), and ibuprofen were used as polymer, emulsifier agent and model drug, respectively. The optimized formulation variables and process parameters for preparing ibuprofen-loaded NP at laboratory scale were selected considering the findings reported in previous studies (Galindo-Rodriguez et al., 2004a,b).

2. Materials and methods

2.1. Materials

Ibuprofen was a gift from Laboratoires UPSA (Rueil-Malmaison, France). Poly(vinyl alcohol), with a molecular weight of 26 000 and a hydrolysis degree of 88% (Mowiol$^®$ 4-88), was kindly supplied by Omya AG (Oftringen, Switzerland). Methacrylic acid copolymer Type C USP/NF (Eudragit$^®$ L 100-

55) was a gift from Röhm GmbH & Co. KG (Darmstadt, Germany). All other chemicals used were of reagent grade.

2.2. Procedures for nanoparticle production

Nanoparticles were prepared according to standard procedures of the salting-out (Bindschaedler et al., 1988), emulsification-diffusion (Leroux et al., 1995) and nanoprecipitation (Fessi et al., 1989) methods. Modifications of these general procedures (Fig. 1) will be detailed in the Results and Discussion sections. In all cases, scale-up was achieved by increasing 20-fold the materials used for the lab-scale batches. Table 1 presents the exact composition of the aqueous and organic phases used for the three methods.

2.2.1. Salting-out
For the lab-scale, 50 g of an aqueous solution were added under mechanical stirring (Eurostar digital stirrer, IKA, Staufen, Germany) to 30 g of an organic phase. Agitation was maintained at the required stirring rate for 15 min. After emulsification, 50 g of pure water were added to induce the diffusion of the organic solvent into the external phase and the formation of NP. The dimensions of the agitation systems used for the emulsification step are shown in Table 2. For the pilot-scale experiments, 1000 g of aqueous phase, 600 g of organic phase and 1000 g of pure water were used.

2.2.2. Emulsification-diffusion
For the lab-scale, 40 g of an aqueous solution were added under stirring to 21 g of an organic solution. The resulting o/w emulsion was stirred continuously for 15 min. Then, 660 g of water were introduced in order to allow the diffusion of

the organic solvent into the water, leading to NP formation. Emulsification was performed using the same agitation system as that for salting-out. Scale-up for this method was carried out using 800 g of aqueous phase, 420 g of organic phase and 13 200 g of pure water.

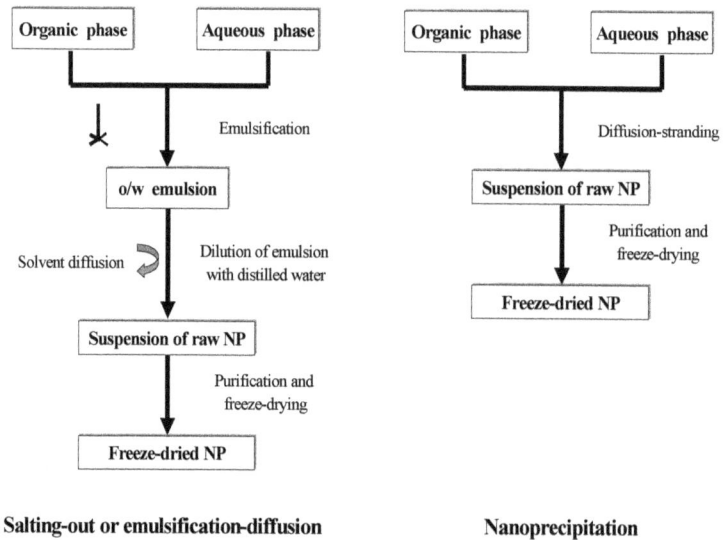

Salting-out or emulsification-diffusion   **Nanoprecipitation**

Fig. 1. General procedures of nanoparticle preparation.

Table 1. Compositions (%, w/w) of the aqueous and organic phases used in the salting-out, emulsification-diffusion and nanoprecipitation methods

Formulation	Salting-out	Emulsification-diffusion	Nanoprecipitation
Organic phase			
Eudragit® L 100-55	9.0	14.3	1.44
Ibuprofen	1.0	1.4	0.14
Organic solvent	90.0 [a]	84.3 [b]	100.00 [a]
Aqueous phase			
Mowiol® 4-88	9.0	12.0	0.8
Mg Cl$_2$ · 6H$_2$O	34.0	-----	-----
HCl conc. q.s.	pH = 1.5	pH = 1.5	-----
Distilled water	57.0	88.0	50.0

[a] Acetone was used for salting-out and nanoprecipitation.
[b] Benzyl alcohol was used for emulsification-diffusion.

Table 2. Main characteristics of the laboratory and pilot agitation systems used in the emulsification step of the salting-out and emulsification-diffusion methods

Characteristics	Lab-scale	Pilot-scale
Reactor capacity [a] (l)	0.2	2.0
Reactor internal diameter [a] (m)	0.07	0.15
Volume of the emulsion (l)		
Salting-out	0.076	1.528
Emulsification-diffusion	0.059	1.173
Impeller diameter [b] (m)	0.04	0.08
Number of baffles	-----	4
Stirring rate (rpm)	790 – 2000	790 – 2000

[a] This corresponds to R-2 in Fig. 2.
[b] 45° pitched blade turbine.

55

Chapitre III

2.2.3. Pilot-scale production of the emulsion-based methods

The equipment used for pilot-scale production was composed of three double jacketed reactors which can be connected depending on the requirements of each fabrication process. The characteristics (dimensions) of the main reactor, in which the emulsification step is performed (R-2 in Fig.2), are presented in Table 2. This reactor had a total capacity of 2 l and was equipped with four baffles. Its content was stirred (Eurostar power control-visc stirrer, IKA-WERKE, Staufen, Germany) with a 45° pitched blade turbine. The characteristics of the other reactors are mentioned in Fig. 2. The experimental set-up for the salting-out (Fig. 2-A) and emulsification diffusion (Fig. 2-B) methods will also be described in the discussion of results.

The flow of the products from one reactor to another was enabled by gravity. Stirring rate (790 ≤ N ≤ 2000 rpm), in a range generally corresponding to a turbulent flow regime, was the parameter evaluated for the two methods at both scales. The flow regime for each emulsified system was determined considering the dimensionless Reynolds number (Re) which was calculated from Eq (1):

$$Re = \rho_c N D^2 / \eta_c \qquad (1)$$

where N is the stirring rate (s^{-1}), D is the impeller diameter (m), ρ_c is the specific gravity of the continuous phase (kg/m^3) and η_c is the viscosity of the continuous phase (Pa·s). Experimental values of N, D, ρ_c and η_c are reported in Table 2 and Table 3. As shown in Table 4, most of the emulsions were prepared under a turbulent flow regime (Re ≥ 10^4). Only a few emulsions produced at lab-scale for the salting-out method (from 790 to 1250 rpm) had a Re that was slightly lower than 10^4. However, because of the negligible difference, the few regimens can be considered to be turbulent in nature.

2.2.4. Nanoprecipitation

For the lab-scale (Fig. 1), the organic solution (25 ml) was added to the aqueous phase (50 ml) containing the stabilizing agent and stirred magnetically. The solvent was then evaporated under reduced pressure. For the pilot-scale, the required volumes of the organic and aqueous phases were 500 and 1000 ml, respectively.

A) Salting-out

B) Emulsification-diffusion

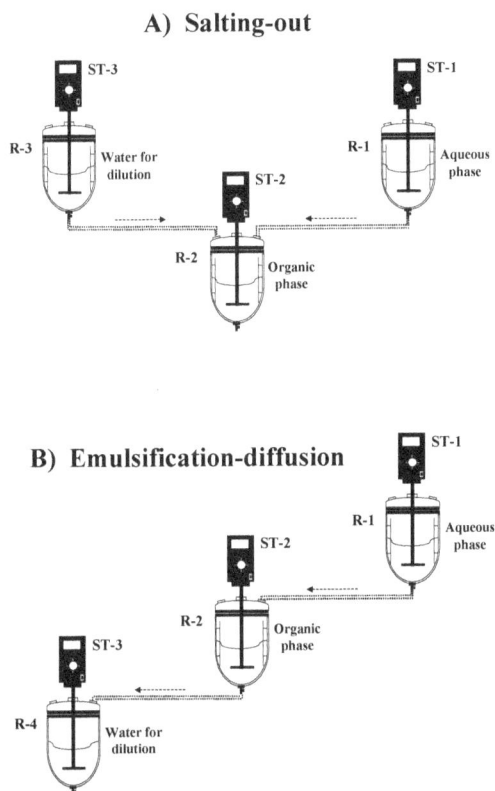

Fig. 2. Set-up for the scaling-up of the two emulsion-based methods. Abbreviations: ST-1, ST-2 and ST-3, stirrers (Eurostar power control-visc stirrer, IKA-WERKE, Staufen, Germany); R-1, 2.5 l reactor; R-2, 2.0 l reactor; R-3, 2 l reactor; R-4, 15 l reactor; all stirred reactors were equipped with four baffles and agitated with a 45° pitched blade turbine; only for R-4 baffles were excluded.

Table 3. Physicochemical properties [a] of the fluids involved in the preparation of nanoparticles by the salting-out and emulsification-diffusion methods

Property	Salting-out			Emulsification-diffusion		
	Aqueous phase	Organic phase	Emulsion	Aqueous phase	Organic phase	Emulsion
Viscosity (Pa·s) [b]	0.119	0.012	0.075	0.039	2.177	0.545
Density (g/ml) [c]	1.161	0.812	1.047	1.024	1.066	1.040
Interfacial tension (mN/m) [d]	-----	-----	1.34 [e]	-----	-----	2.44 [e]
Surface tension (mN/m) [d]	44.8	24.8	-----	42.6	39.8	-----

[a] All measurements were performed in triplicate at 25 °C.
[b] Viscometer Contraves mod. Rheomat 15 T, Zurich, Switzerland.
[c] Pycnometer, 10.08 ml capacity.
[d] Tensiometer Krüss model K12, Krüss GmbH, Hamburg, Germany.
[e] Interfacial tension between the aqueous and organic phases.

Table 4. Calculated Reynolds number (Re) [a] for emulsified systems formed during NP preparation by the salting-out and emulsification-diffusion methods.

Stirring rate (rpm)	$Re_{salting-out}$ ($\times 10^{-4}$)		$Re_{emulsification-diffusion}$ ($\times 10^{-4}$)	
	Lab-scale	Pilot-scale	Lab-scale	Pilot-scale
2000	1.3	2.6	3.5	7.0
1750	1.1	2.3	3.1	6.1
1500	1.0	2.0	2.6	5.3
1250	0.8	1.6	2.2	4.4
1000	0.7	1.3	1.8	3.5
790	0.5	1.0	1.4	2.8

[a] Re was calculated from Eq (1) using experimental data from Tables 2 and 3.

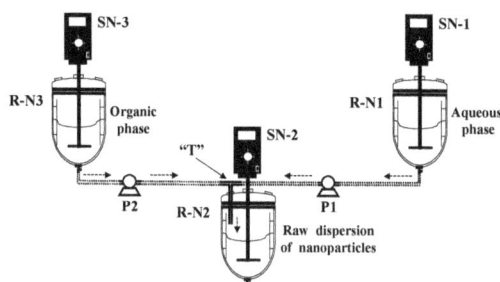

Fig. 3. Set-up for the scaling-up of the nanoprecipitation method. Abbreviations: SN-1, SN-2 and SN-3, stirrers (RW 20DZW.n stirrer, IKA-Labortechnik, Staufen, Germany); R-N1, R-N2 and R-N3, 2.5 1 reactors equipped with four baffles and an axial impeller; P1 and P2, peristaltic pumps; T, "Tee mixer".

2.2.5. Pilot-scale production of the nanoprecipitation method

The scale-up for this technique was performed using a continuous method which has been well characterized and optimised previously {Briancon et. al., 1999}. A schematic diagram of the experimental set-up is shown in Fig. 3. This consists of three reactors (R-N1, R-N2, R-N3) each equipped with an axial impeller. The R-N1 and R-N3 reservoirs contain the aqueous and organic phases, respectively. Both phases are continuously supplied by independent peristaltic pumps (P1 and P2). The interesting point of this continuous system is a "Tee mixer" which serves to mix the two phases. In fact, when both phases come into contact in the central part of the "Tee mixer", they diffuse into each other forming immediately the NP. The raw NP dispersion is finally received in the main reactor (R-N2) and maintained under a gentle agitation.

For the three methods, raw NP were separated from free surfactant and solvent by centrifugation (Centrifuge model Avanti 30, Beckman Instruments, California, U.S.A.). Briefly, a sample of raw NP dispersion (60 g) was washed twice using 30 ml of water adjusted to pH = 3.0 with HCl and finally with deionised water. After recovery, the washed NP were freeze-dried (LSL Secfroid, model Lyolab BII, Switzerland).

2.3. Characterization of nanoparticles

2.3.1. Analysis of nanoparticle mean size
The mean size and polydispersity of raw NP dispersions were assessed by photon correlation spectroscopy (Zetasizer 3000®, Malvern Instruments, Worcestershire, U.K.). With respect to the polydispersity index (P.I.), which ranges from 0 to 1, a higher value corresponds to a less homogeneous NP size distribution.

2.3.2. Drug loading
Samples of freeze-dried NP were accurately weighed and dissolved in 0.1 N NaOH. The ibuprofen content was determined spectrophotometrically at $\lambda_{max} =$ 272 nm (Hewlett Packard 8453 Spectrophotometer, Germany). Three samples were examined for three different batches of each NP formulation.

2.3.3. Residual PVAL

Nanoparticles were assayed for residual PVAL using a method that involves the formation of a stable complex of PVAL with iodine in presence of boric acid (Allémann et al., 1993). First, freeze-dried NP were dissolved in 0.1 M NaOH. Subsequently, Eudragit L100-55 was precipitated by the addition of 0.1 M HCl and the suspension centrifuged. Then, an aliquot of supernatant was treated with 7.5 ml of boric acid solution (4.0%, w/v) and 1.5 ml of iodine solution (1.27% iodine and 2.50% potassium iodide in distilled water, w/v), and the volume adjusted to 25.0 ml with water. Finally, the absorbance was measured at 644 nm.

2.3.4. Scanning electron microscopy

Morphological examination of NP was performed using a scanning electron microscope (model JEOL JSM-6400, Jeol Ltd., Japan). Samples of dried NP were dispersed in water, and then drops of the dispersion were placed on metallic studs and coated with gold.

2.4. Characterization of the fluids involved in the emulsion-based methods

2.4.1. Viscosity

The viscosity of the aqueous phases, organic phases and emulsions, prepared for the salting-out and emulsification-diffusion methods, was determined at 25 °C using a cone-plate system (Viscometer Contraves, Rheomat 15 T, Zurich, Switzerland). Each determination was made in triplicate.

2.4.2. Surface and interfacial tensions

The plate method was used for surface and interfacial tension determinations (Digital Tensiometer K12, Krüss, Hamburg, Germany). Each measurement was made in triplicate at 25 °C.

2.4.3. Density

Density measurements were carried out using a picnometer. Each determination was performed in triplicate at 25 °C.

3. Results and discussion

3.1. Preparation of nanoparticles by the emulsion-based methods

During NP preparation using the emulsion-based methods, such as salting-out and emulsification-diffusion, a nanoemulsion is formed due to dispersion of an organic phase into an aqueous phase by shear mixing. After emulsification, water is added to the emulsion in order to remove the solvent from the droplets and induce NP formation. At that point, it has been established that NP features, such as size, are determined by the characteristics of the precursor nanoemulsion (Galindo-Rodriguez et al., 2004a; Lemarchand et al., 2003). This fact is of great importance because the final droplet size of a liquid-liquid dispersion in agitated vessels depends on parameters such as the physicochemical characteristics of the two phases (e.g. viscosity, interfacial tension, stabilizer concentration), the preparation conditions of the emulsion (e.g. temperature, addition order of the components) and the agitation system (e.g. shear rate, design of the stirrer and containing vessel). In particular, because one of the major problems in the transition from lab-scale to pilot-scale is to provide similar hydrodynamic conditions, the first part of this study focused on determining the effect of stirring rate on the NP mean size.

3.1.1. Lab-scale production

Nanoparticles were produced according to salting-out and emulsification procedures. Although both preparation techniques are quite similar (Fig. 1), the dilution-diffusion step is slightly different. Whilst pure water is added to the emulsion for salting-out, the emulsion is incorporated into water for emulsification-diffusion. In the first case, this is technically possible because the reactor containing the emulsion is large enough to accommodate the water. In contrast, for the second case, because a much larger volume of water is needed for dilution (600 ml) and the reactor capacity is limited to 200 ml, the emulsion has to be transferred to a larger reactor which contains the pure water for dilution. As illustrated in Fig. 4, NP mean size decreases on increasing the stirring rate. For salting-out, mean sizes of NP from 719 to 279 nm were obtained when the stirring rate was varied from 790 to 2000 rpm. In emulsification-diffusion, for the same range of stirring rate, NP mean sizes ranged from 421 to 300 nm. This can be explained considering that, in a stirred vessel, the mean droplet size of an emulsion system is governed by the balance between the break-up and coalescence of droplets. These phenomena occur simultaneously during emulsification, so their relative kinetics determine the final droplet size. The maximum diameter of the emulsion droplets is linked to the break-up mechanism whereas the minimum diameter depends on the coalescence phenomenon (Baldyga et al., 2001). Likewise, the breakage forces depend on the power input per unit mass, which increases by increasing the stirring speed. Therefore, the droplet break-up process increases with the stirring speed leading to formation of finer emulsion droplets, and thus smaller NP.

On the other hand, for a given stirring rate, particle size was generally reproducible. Very similar results were obtained from three separate batches as attested by the low standard deviation values (S.D. in Fig. 4). This also shows that the mixing efficiency was acceptable. However, at stirring rates ≤ 790 rpm for salting-out and ≤ 1000 rpm for emulsification diffusion, raw NP dispersions were heterogeneous in their size distribution and exhibited the presence of particles larger than 1 μm (batches marked with [*] in Fig. 4). These findings revealed that break-up efficiency decreased, while the coalescence process was favoured, when the stirring rate was reduced.

3.1.2. Pilot-scale production

Scale-up production for emulsion-based methods was carried out by increasing 20-fold the volume of the laboratory batches. For salting-out, the set-up is illustrated in Fig. 2-A. Geometric similarities of the agitation systems used at lab- and pilot- scales for the emulsification step (Table 2) were maintained as much as possible in order to obtain a similar fluid motion at both scales. Briefly, the organic phase was first introduced in R-2, and the aqueous phase was then added from R-1 by gravity. After 30 min of emulsification, the pure water contained in R-3 was incorporated. Agitation was maintained for 5 min.

For emulsification-diffusion, because of the large volume of water used for the dilution step, the configuration of the reactors previously used for salting-out was changed. The third reactor was substituted with another (R-4) of a larger capacity (15 l). The experimental set-up used for this technique is shown in Fig. 2-B. Under these conditions, it was possible to reproduce the lab-scale procedure.

A) Salting-out

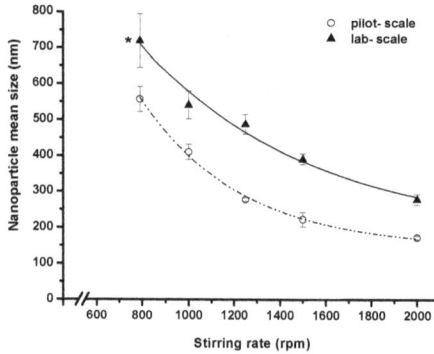

B) Emulsification-diffusion

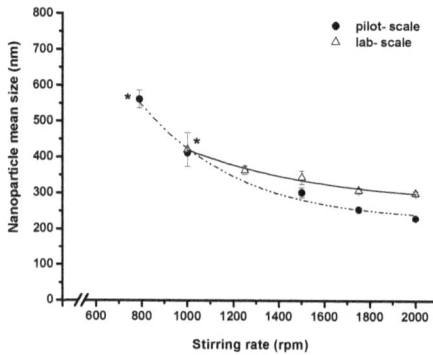

Fig. 4. Influence of stirring rate on the mean size of nanoparticles prepared by salting-out and emulsification-diffusion at the laboratory and pilot scales. An abundant presence of particles larger than 1 μm was found in batches marked with *. (Mean ± S.D., n=3)

Chapitre III

The aqueous phase contained in R-1 was added to R-2 containing the organic phase. Stirring was maintained for 30 min. Afterwards, the emulsion was transferred into R-4 which had previously contained the pure water intended for the dilution-diffusion step. During introduction of the emulsion, R-4 was gently stirred.

As expected, when increasing the agitation rate, the NP mean size clearly shifted to smaller diameters (Fig. 4). The NP mean sizes varied from 557 to 174 nm for salting-out and from 562 to 230 nm for emulsification-diffusion when the stirring rate changed from 790 to 2000 rpm. It was also noted that, for stirring rates $\geq$ 1000 rpm reasonably narrow size distributions were obtained which, in turn, revealed that uniform emulsification processes were achieved. However, below 1000 rpm for emulsification-diffusion and 790 rpm for salting-out, the high values of the standard deviation (S.D. in Fig. 4) show that batch to batch reproducibility was severely affected, which may be attributed to a heterogeneous dispersion of the organic liquid phase. In those cases, the insufficient energy input supplied by the stirrer as well as the high viscosity of the external phase led to a decrease in emulsification break-up efficiency thus favouring droplet coalescence. This results in +heterogeneous size distributions for the individual batches which systematically exhibited the presence of a high number of particles larger than 1 μm (batches marked with [*] in Fig. 4). Obviously, a lack of homogeneity of the individual batches leads to high differences when inter-batch comparisons are made.

When comparing the curves obtained at the lab- and pilot- scales, it is observed that the patterns are quite similar in the salting-out method and emulsification-diffusion methods (Fig. 4), which indicates that the break-up and coalescence processes were reproduced with the agitation systems employed at both scales.

3.1.3. Theoretical considerations for modeling the emulsion-based methods
In the literature, mathematical models for the formation of NP produced by salting out and emulsion diffusion are not yet established. Because in both processes the size of NP is determined by the size of the precursor nanoemulsion, it is convenient to consider a model for describing the formation of the droplets in the nanoemulsion.

Here, we present a classical theory used for modeling dispersed liquid-liquid systems in stirred vessels originating from the chemical engineering field (Baldyga et al., 2001). Although this theory has been developed for emulsions in the micrometric size range, some authors have recently attempted to apply it to the case of nanoemulsion systems (Rivautella et al., 2003). In that study, the mean nanoparticle size was calculated assuming that each nanodroplet leads to one nanoparticle and considering that the nanodroplets and the nanoparticles are not porous.

The phenomenon of droplet dispersion has been studied by many researchers based on the fundamental papers by Kolmogorov (1949) and Hinze (1955). The theory of local isotropic turbulence applicable to a dispersed phase gives a relationship between the maximum stable drop size of the droplets (d_{max}, m) and the stirring rate (N, s^{-1}), the stirrer diameter (D, m), the interfacial tension (σ, Nm) and the specific gravity of the continuous phase (ρ_c, kg/m^3):

$$d_{max} \propto N^{-6/5} D^{-4/5} \sigma^{3/5} \rho_c^{-3/5} \qquad (2)$$

Because it is not possible to measure the maximum stable drop size, the d_{max} is often substituted by the surface-volume mean diameter (Sauter diameter). Likewise, when the Sauter diameter is not known, a mean volume diameter is also accepted. It should be also noted that the Eq (2) is mainly valid if the hydrodynamic flow regime is turbulent. As discussed in section 2.2.3., most of the systems analyzed in this study satisfied this condition.

Depending on the parameter to be studied, other equivalent expressions of the relationship (2) can be found in the literature. As shown in Eq (3), the dimensionless Weber number (We) can be introduced in order to estimate the size of the emulsion droplets ($d_{mean\ drop}$). Thus:

$$\frac{d_{mean\ drop}}{D} \propto We^{-3/5} \propto \left[\frac{\sigma}{N^2 D^3 \rho_c}\right]^{3/5} \qquad (3)$$

This equation has been shown to fit experimental data by many workers (Chen and Middleman, 1967; Calabrese et al., 1986). Numerous correlations depending on the type of the stirrer and on the physicochemical characteristics of the emulsion have been established (Costaz, 1996).

3.1.3.1. Modeling the effect of the stirring rate on the nanoparticle mean size.-
From Eq (3), it is possible to express the evolution of the droplet mean size with the stirring rate as follows:

$$d_{mean\ drop} = K_2 \left(\frac{\rho_c}{\sigma}\right)^{-0.6} D^{-0.8} N^{-1.2} \qquad (4)$$

where K_2 is a constant. Moreover, for the case of emulsioned systems prepared at the same scale (where D, ρ_c, and σ are constant), Eq (4) can be reduced as following:

$$d_{mean\,drop} = K_3\,N^{-1.2} \tag{5}$$

or in a logarithmic form:

$$\log\,d_{mean\,drop} = \log\,K_3 - 1.2\,\log\,N \tag{5'}$$

where K_3 is a constant. Due to the instability of the nanoemulsion formed during NP preparation by the salting-out and emulsification-diffusion methods, it was not possible to determine the size distribution of the droplets of the emulsion. Nevertheless, as mentioned above, one can assume (a) that each emulsion droplet leads to the formation of one nanoparticle, and (b) that the droplet and the particles are non-porous. Experimental evidence of the first assumption was reported in a previous study (Galindo-Rodriguez et al., 2004a). So, Eq (5) can be represented as follows:

$$d_{mean\,drop} \propto d_{mean\,nanoparticle} \propto N^{-1.2} \tag{6}$$

where $d_{mean\,nanoparticle}$ corresponds to the mean size of nanoparticles.

The logarithmic relationship between the stirring rate and the mean size of nanoparticles obtained by the salting-out and emulsification-diffusion methods is plotted in Fig. 5, at both lab- and pilot- scales. Each series of data was fitted using a linear relationship where the slope (*m*) of the curves corresponded to the exponent of Eq (6). At pilot-scale, the experimental values obtained for salting-out (-1.3) and for emulsification-diffusion (-0.9) were quite close to the

71

theoretical one (-1.2) which indicates that this model can adequately describe the influence of stirring rate on the nanoparticle mean size. Other authors have found a similar behavior for emulsified systems in the micrometer range (Jégat and Taverdet, 2000). In contrast, two situations might be observed at lab-scale. While the value of the slope obtained from the salting-out method (-1.0) was considered as correct, the value resulting from emulsification-diffusion (-0.5) showed a significant difference compared to the theoretical value (-1.2). This discrepancy could have multiple origins. For instance, it is suspected that the stirring configuration was not well-defined at lab-scale (e.g. the absence of baffles). However, since this factor is not sufficient to explain the deviations at lab-scale, other unknown factors have to be investigated in further studies.

Based on the pilot-scale results, it might be concluded that the tested model, usually applied to liquid-liquid dispersions sized in the micrometer range and having a low volume fraction of dispersed phase, was suitable for predicting the effect of stirring speed on the NP mean size.

3.1.3.2. Modeling the effect of scale-up on the mean size of nanoparticles.- The important concept for scale-up in chemical engineering science is the principle of similarity. In the case of the emulsions prepared in stirred vessels, the following three types of similarity need to be considered: geometric, kinematic, and dynamic. Two systems are geometrically similar when the ratio of the linear dimensions of the small scale vessel and scale-up vessel is constant. Kinematics similarity means that the fluid motion in a vessel is similar for both scales and is provided when the relative geometry of the vessel is maintained (Letellier et al., 2002).

A) Salting-out

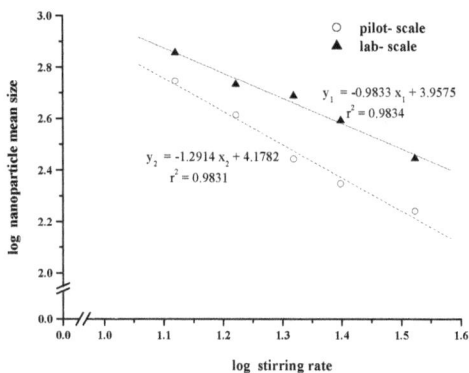

B) Emulsification-diffusion

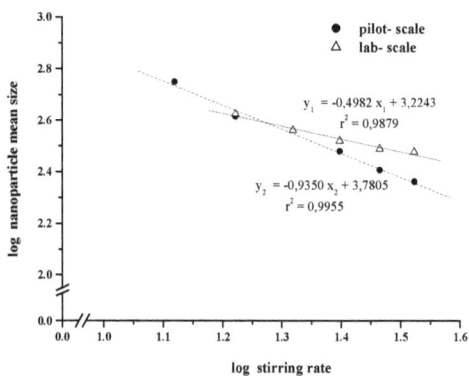

Fig. 5. Logarithmic relationship between the stirring rate and diameter of nanoparticles (Eq 5') prepared, at lab- and pilot- scales, by the salting-out and emulsification-diffusion methods. The slope of the curves also corresponds to exponent of N in Eq (6).

73

Finally, two systems of different size are dynamically similar when in addition to their geometric and kinematic similarities, the ratio of forces between corresponding points in the two systems are equal. This is obtained when a representative criterion is kept constant. In the case of the emulsification process, the specific power input of the stirrer (ε) is employed. ε is the ratio of the power (P) imparted by the stirring to the volume (V) of the emulsion. ε can also be expressed in relation to the stirring speed (N) and the diameter of the stirrer (D) as :

$$\varepsilon = \frac{P}{V} \propto N^3 D^2 \tag{7}$$

Subsequently, the combination of the Eqs (2) and (7) gives the following expression:

$$d_{mean\text{-}drop} \propto \varepsilon^{-2/5} \left(\frac{\sigma}{\rho_c} \right)^{3/5} \tag{8}$$

Because Eq (8) is valid for both scales, during the scale-up process it should be attempted to closely reproduce $\varepsilon_{pilot\text{-}}$ and $\varepsilon_{lab\text{-}}$ in order to obtain similar mean sizes of emulsion droplets at pilot- and lab- scales. In Fig. 6, the evolution of the mean diameter of the particles is plotted versus ε. As the batch volume increases, the mean size of NP shifts to smaller values . This drift indicates that the break-up phenomena is increased with the size of the batch, leading to smaller droplets in larger stirred tanks. In conclusion, scale up induces smaller nanoparticles.

A) Salting-out

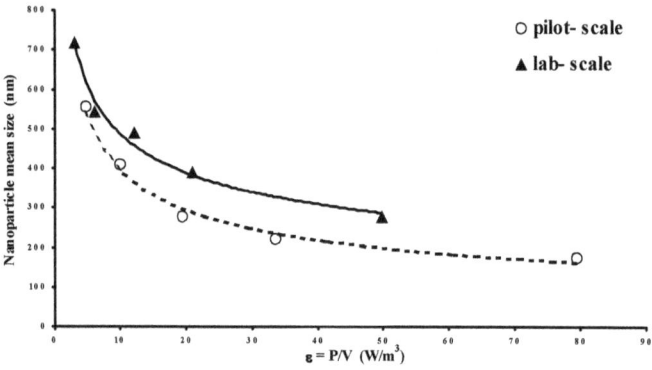

B) Emulsification-diffusion

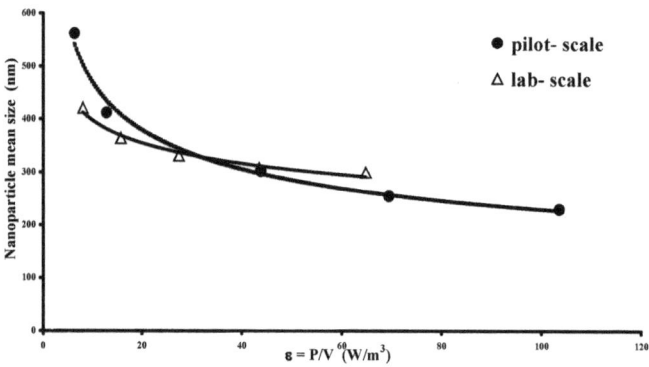

Fig. 6. Relationship between the specific power input of the stirrer and the nanoparticle mean size.

This effect of scale-up on the droplet size of liquid-liquid turbulent dispersion has been already observed and widely discussed for emulsions in the micrometric range (Baldyga et al., 2001). However, in this study we have demonstrated that the same trend can also be encountered for emulsion systems in the nanometric size range.

3.2. Laboratory and pilot production of nanoparticles by the nanoprecipitation method

Nanoparticle formation during the nanoprecipitation method is governed by the "diffusion-stranding phenomena". In the early stage of this process, the solvent and polymer chains contained in the organic phase together diffuse into the continuous aqueous phase. Later, further diffusion of the solvent induces the desolvation of polymer chains which aggregate to form NP. As shown in other studies (Galindo-Rodriguez et al., 2004a), any change in the solvent-diffusion behaviour leads to changes in the NP mean size. The characteristics of the aqueous and organic phases as well as the general procedure used in this study can be seen in Table 1 and Fig. 1, respectively.

Nanoparticles produced at lab-scale manifested homogeneous populations characterized by their narrow size distributions. The NP mean size corresponded to 141 ± 5 nm (Mean ± S.D., n=3). In particular, the S.D. shows a low batch to batch variability. At pilot-scale, a continuous method (Fig. 3) was employed to prepare NP of reproducible sizes. The organic phase and aqueous phase were mixed in a ratio of 1:2 (v:v) by adjusting their flow rates to 62.5 and 125.0 ml/min, respectively. Under these conditions, average particle diameters of 105 ± 8 nm and reasonably narrow size distributions were systematically obtained. A systematic difference (~ 35 nm) in NP diameter was observed between the lab- and pilot- batches, which may be attributed to differences in the hydrodynamic conditions generated in the course of each manufacturing process. At lab-scale, NP are prepared by a batch system in which organic phase is poured into the aqueous phase under magnetic agitation. In contrast, at pilot-scale, NP production is performed using a continuous system in which turbulence of the external phase is more pronounced. Since NP formation in the nanoprecipitation process depends on the diffusion of the solvent contained in the organic phase (Galindo-Rodriguez et al., 2003a), it is probable that the higher turbulence generated may improve the diffusion of solvent and hence the partition of the polymer chains into the aqueous phase, which would ultimately induce the formation of smaller NP. In general, the continuous method used for nanoprecipitation was the simplest scale-up process for producing NP. Moreover, pilot batches demonstrated good inter-batch reproducibility and required only 120 min to produce each batch (see section 3.4.). However, as already stated, the main drawback of this method was related to the low polymer concentration in the organic phase, which significantly limits the NP recovery in the final raw dispersion.

3.3. Influence of the scale-up process on the characteristics of nanoparticles: drug loading, residual PVAL and morphology

In order to determine the effect of hydrodynamic conditions of the scale-up process on NP characteristics, NP of similar size were prepared at the lab- and pilot- scales and they were compared in terms of their drug loading, residual PVAL and morphology. For the emulsion based methods, stirring rate was adjusted in order to obtain NP with a mean size of around 300 nm. In salting-

77

out, although NP showed similar mean sizes (Table 5), lab-scale NP exhibited higher drug loading than those prepared by pilot-scale. These corresponded to 8.8 and 7.5%, respectively. A similar trend was observed in the emulsification-diffusion method: lab-scale and pilot-scale batches had drug loadings of 7.7% and 5.5%, respectively. These findings suggest that the scale-up process slightly influence the drug loading of NP. In contrast, residual PVAL was found to be unaffected by the scale-up process (Table 5): the percentage of residual PVAL in batches prepared at lab- and pilot- scales was practically the same. This can be explained on the basis of the mechanism of interaction of PVAL at the emulsion droplet interface and the NP mean size. It has been established that, during the emulsification and solvent diffusion steps of NP preparation, PVAL chains remain on the NP even after several washing cycles, essentially due to physical binding at the droplet interface between the PVAL and the polymer chains contained in the internal organic phase (Galindo-Rodriguez et al., 2004a).

Table 5. Comparison of the nanoparticles prepared at the laboratory and pilot scales (Mean ± S.D., n=3)

Nanoparticle characteristics [a]	Salting-out		Emulsification-diffusion		Nanoprecipitation	
	Lab-scale	Pilot-scale	Lab-scale	Pilot-scale	Lab-scale	Pilot-scale
Mean diameter (nm)	274 ± 15	281 ± 5	293 ± 15	287 ± 12	141 ± 5	105 ± 8
Polydispersity index [b] (0-1)	0.085 ± 0.012	0.091 ± 0.005	0.082 ± 0.021	0.116 ± 0.027	0.082 ± 0.023	0.130 ± 490
Ibuprofen loading (%)	8.8 ± 0.3	7.5 ± 0.4	7.7 ± 0.2	5.5 ± 0.3	4.5 ± 0.3	3.2 ± 0.4
Entrapment efficiency [c] (%)	88	75	86	62	50	39
Residual PVAL (%)	5.6 ± 0.1	5.5 ± 0.4	4.8 ± 0.2	5.0 ± 0.1	3.7 ± 0.3	4.0 ± 0.4

[a] Three determinations were made for three different batches.
[b] For polydispersity index (P.I.), which ranges from 0 to 1, a higher value correspond to less homogeneous particle size distribution.
[c] Entrapment efficiency was the ratio of the experimentally measured ibuprofen content and the theoretical value expressed as a percentage.

Since NP prepared by lab- and pilot- scales had similar mean size and specific surface area, the number of PVAL chains that can be adsorbed onto the NP will also be the same. As a result, residual PVAL values are similar. Finally, scanning electron micrographs of freeze dried NP, prepared at the lab-scale and pilot-scale, are shown in Fig. 7.

Laboratory scale Pilot scale

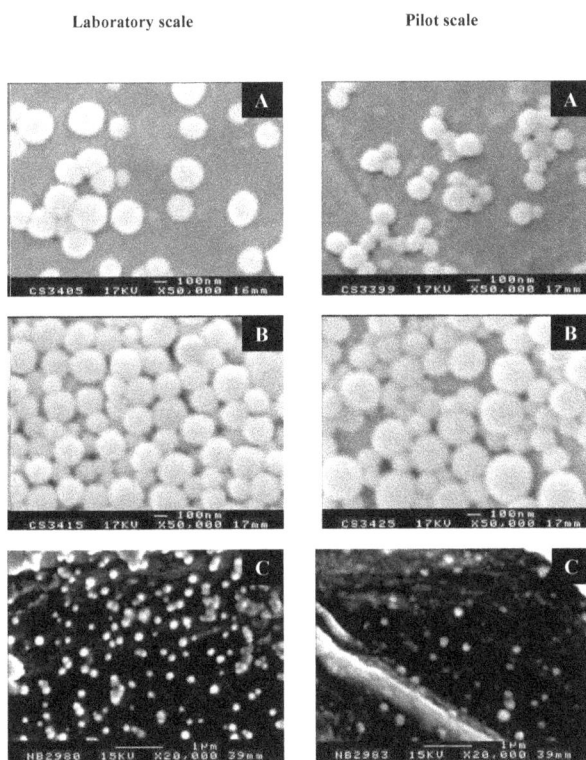

Fig. 7. Scanning electron micrographs of nanoparticles prepared, at laboratory and pilot scales, by A) emulsification-diffusion, B) salting-out and C) nanoprecipitation.

In the emulsification-diffusion method, although NP are not totally spherical (Fig. 7-A), they appear to be homogeneous in size. The lack of roundness is probably due to the application of a vacuum during the freeze drying stage. For salting-out, micrographs (Fig. 7-B) showed spherical NP of sub-300 nm diameter with a relatively homogeneous size distribution. These results indicate that NP with similar morphological characteristics can be produced at both, lab- and pilot- scales.

In general, although this first approach can be considered acceptable, further studies should be conducted in order to optimize the scale-up processes of the emulsion-based methods. Considering differences in the drug loading, special attention should be paid to other influential variables such as the hydrodynamic conditions of the dilution step as well as the thermal similarity of the whole process.

For the nanoprecipitation method, ibuprofen loading was significantly higher for the NP prepared at lab-scale (4.5 %) than for those produced at pilot-scale (3.2 %). This can be explained by differences in the "diffusion-stranding" phenomena of both systems. The higher turbulence in the continuous mode could have induced diffusion of the drug into the external aqueous phase before aggregation of the polymer chains to form the NP. Finally, the scanning electron microscopy analysis revealed the presence of spherical structures of around 100 nm for the pilot-scale and 100-140 nm for the lab-scale (Fig. 7-C). In both cases, the particle size distribution was reasonably homogeneous.

3.4. Time consumption for the three scale-up processes

Finally, the time taken by each technique to produce a single pilot-batch was also determined. The estimation was made by considering all operations involved from the preparation of raw solutions (aqueous and organic phases) to the formation of the raw NP dispersion (Fig. 8). It was noted that producing a pilot-batch by salting-out required less time (300 min) compared to emulsification-diffusion (350 min). Nevertheless, the shortest consumption time corresponded to the nanoprecipitation process, i.e. 120 min.

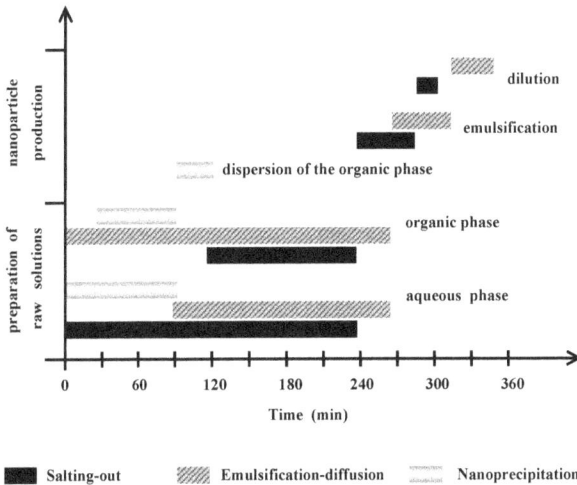

Fig. 8 Time consumption for producing a pilot-batch of nanoparticles by salting-out, emulsification-diffusion and nanoprecipitation.

Figure 8 also illustrates that for the emulsion-based methods, the preparation of raw solutions is the critical step because it consumes more that 60 % of the global production time. This is because high amounts of polymer, PVAL in the aqueous phase and Eudragit® L100-55 in the organic phase, have to be dissolved in the raw solutions (Table 1). However, this is not completely unfavourable because a high polymer content in the organic phase enables a high recovery of NP in the final raw dispersion. Considering the composition of the organic phases for each method, 169.6, 100.0 and 18.0 mg of NP per g of organic solvent can be potentially obtained by emulsification-diffusion, salting-out and nanoprecipitation, respectively. Clearly, the two higher theoretical NP recoveries correspond to the emulsion-based methods.

4. Conclusions

This study shows that the scale-up of ibuprofen-loaded NP prepared by the salting-out, emulsification-diffusion and nanoprecipitation methods is feasible. However, certain parameters of each scaled-up method should be considered in order to achieve more favourable results.

By increasing the stirring rate, the mean size of nanoparticles can be systematically varied from 557 to 174 nm and from 562 to 230 nm for the pilot-batches prepared by salting-out and emulsification-diffusion, respectively. An increase in the stirring rate enhances the droplet break-up phenomenon which leads to the formation of finer emulsion droplets and thus smaller NP.

A well known model used in the chemical engineering field was used for modeling the emulsification step of the two emulsion-based methods. This model, which is usually applied to liquid-liquid dispersions sized in the micrometer range and having a low volume fraction of dispersed phase, enables prediction of the NP mean size from the stirring rate. The accuracy of the model is better at pilot-scale (few liters).

Moreover, the scale-up method is based on preserving similarities. When the classical criterion (namely the specific power input of stirring) used in emulsification is kept constant at both lab- and pilot- scales, the NP sizes are not constant. Larger scales of a few liters induce smaller NP sizes.

With respect to the nanoprecipitation method, the continuous mode used for its scale-up allows production of NP in a facile and reproducible way. This method enables the preparation of batches of different volumes, from some milliliters to several liters, only by adjusting very few process parameters (e.g. flow rates of the organic and aqueous phase). Compared to the emulsion-based methods, less time is required for preparing a pilot-batch. However, the drawback of this method was the low polymer concentration in the organic phase which leads to a poor NP yield in the final raw dispersion.

Finally, it can be concluded that pilot-scale production of ibuprofen-loaded NP, prepared by salting-out, emulsification-diffusion and nanoprecipitation, was relatively well achieved. In general, NP characteristics – drug loading, residual PVAL and morphology –were reproduced at lab- and pilot- scales. However, the scale-up process induced a slight reduction in the size and drug loading of NP.

Acknowledges

S. Galindo-Rodriguez was supported by a grant from CONACYT-SFERE (México-France). He also acknowledges FES-Cuautitlan, UNAM, México. The authors are grateful to Mrs C. Siegfried and N. Boulens for their technical assistance in the SEM.

References

Allémann E., Leroux J.C., Gurny R., Doelker, E., 1993. *In vitro* extended-release properties of drug-loaded poly(D,L-lactic acid) nanoparticles produced by a salting-out procedure. Pharm. Res. 10, 1732-1737.

Baldyga J. , Bourne, J.R., Pacek, A.W., Amanullah, A., and Nienow, A.W., 2001. Effects of agitation and scale-up on drop size in turbulent dispersions: allowance for intermittency. Chem. Eng. Sci. 56, 3377-3385.

Bindschaedler, C., Gurny, R., Doelker, E., 1988. Process for preparing a powder of water-insoluble polymer which can be redispersed in a liquid phase, the resulting powder and utilization thereof. Patent WO 88/08011.

Briançon, S., Fessi, H., Lecomte, F., Lieto, J., 1999. Study of an original production process of nanoparticles by precipitation. 2nd European Congress of Chemical Engineering, Montpellier, France.

Calabrese, R.V., Chang, T.P.K., Dang, P.T., 1986. Drop break-up in turbulent stirred tank contactors, Part I. Effect of dispersed phase viscosity. A. I. Ch. E. Journal. 32, 657-666.

Chen, H.T. and Middleman, S., 1967. Drop size distribution in agitated liquid-liquid systems. A. I. Ch. E. Journal. 13, 989-995.

Colombo, A.P., Briançon, S., Lieto, J., Fessi, H., 2001. Project, design, and use of a pilot plant for nanocapsule production. Drug Dev. Ind. Pharm. 27, 1063-1072.

Chapitre III

Costaz H., 1996. Encapsulation d'un principe actif par double emulsion: mise au point d'un procédé de formation de systèmes réservoirs. PhD Thesis 041-96, Université Claude Bernard Lyon 1, France.

De Labouret, A., Thioune, O., Fessi, H., Devissaguet, J.P., and Puisieux, F., 1995. Application of an original process for obtaining colloidal dispersions of some coating polymers: preparation, characterization, industrial scale-up. Drug Dev. Ind. Pharm. 21, 229-241.

Fessi, H., Puisieux, F., Devissaguet, J.P., Ammoury, N., Benita, S., 1989. Nanocapsule formation by interfacial polymer deposition following solvent displacement. Int. J. Pharm. 55, R1-R4.

Galan Valdivia, F.J., Vallet Mas, J.A., Bergamini, M.V.W., 1998. Process of continuous preparation of disperse colloidal systems in the form of nanocapsules or nanoparticles. U.S. Patent 5,705,196.

Galindo-Rodríguez, S., Allémann, E., Fessi, H., Doelker, E., 2004a. Physicochemical parameters associated with nanoparticle formation in the salting-out, emulsification-diffusion and nanoprecipitation methods. Pharm. Res. 21, 1428-1439.

Galindo-Rodríguez, S., Allémann, E., Fessi, H., Doelker, E., 2004b. Versatility of three techniques for preparing nanoparticles of different sizes and drug loadings. Submitted.

Hinze, J.O., 1955. Fundamentals of the hydrodynamic mechanism of splitting in dispersion processes. A. I. Ch. E. Journal. 1, 289-295.

Jégat, C. and Taverdet, J.L., 2000. Stirring speed influence study on the microencapsulation process and on the drug release from microcapsules. Polym. Bull. 44, 345-351.

Kolmogorov, A.N., 1949. Disintegration of drops in turbulent flow. Doklady Akademmi Nauk SSSR. 66, 825-828.

Transposition d'échelle

Lemarchand, C., Couvreur, P., Besnard, M., Costantini, D., Gref, R., 2003. Novel polyester-polysaccharide nanoparticles. Pharm. Res. 20, 1284-1292.

Leroux, J.C., Allémann, E., Doelker, E., Gurny, R., 1995. New approach for the preparation of nanoparticles by an emulsification-diffusion method. Eur. J. Pharm. Biopharm. 41, 14-18.

Letellier, B., Xuereb, C., Swaels, P., Hobbes, P., Bertrand, J., 2002. Scale-up in laminar and transient regimes of a multi-stage stirrer, a CFD approach. Chem. Eng. Sci. 57, 4617-4632.

Rivautella, L., Briançon, S., Puel, F., 2003. Formation of nanocapsules by emulsion-diffusion: prediction of the emulsion size. 4th European Conference of Chemical Engineering, Grenada, Spain.

ENCAPSULATION DE DEUX MOLÉCULES POSSÉDANT UNE ACTIVITÉ ANTICANCÉREUSE DANS DE NANOPARTICULES BIODÉGRADABLES

INCORPORATION OF TWO NOVEL ALDEHYDE DEHYDROGENASE
INHIBITORS INTO BIODEGRADABLE NANOPARTICLES:
FORMULATION STUDIES AND BIOLOGICAL EVALUATION

S. Galindo-Rodríguez [1,2,3], *G.Quash* [4], *E. Allémann* [2], *E. Doelker* [2] *and H. Fessi* [3]

[1] Pharmapeptides, Geneva-Lyon Interuniversity Center, 74166 Archamps, France.

[2] School of Pharmacy, University of Geneva, 1211 Geneva 4, Switzerland.

[3] UMR-CNRS 5007, Faculty of Pharmacy, Claude Bernard University Lyon I, Lyon, France.

[4] Laboratoire d'Immunochimie, Faculté de Médecine Lyon-Sud, France.

1. INTRODUCTION

1.1. Overview

This part of the thesis deals with the encapsulation of two novel aldehyde dehydrogenase (ALDH1) inhibitors into a biodegradable carrier with the aim of developing a parenteral formulation and possibly improving their anti-tumor activity.

This work is the result of a collaboration with the Immunochemistry Laboratory of the Faculty of Medicine Lyon-Sud (France) where Quash et al. have designed and developed a series of ALDH1 inhibitors with potential use in the treatment of cancer. Among the compounds biologically evaluated, DIMATE and MATE have shown remarkable activity against several types of cancer cells. On the basis of these promising results, such ALDH1 inhibitors were recently patented by Quash et al. (see *Section 1.2.*).

As is frequently the case with newly synthesized, biologically active compounds, the ALDH1 inhibitors are not optimized for therapeutic administration. Owing to their hydrophobic character, these compounds were often dissolved in organic solvents for biological investigations. The need for alternative vehicles for the administration of these molecules is therefore evident.

Polymeric nanoparticles have been often used as drug delivery systems for anticancer drugs. In our laboratory, a novel emulsification-evaporation method for the preparation of these colloidal carriers was developed and recently patented. This technique, described in *Section 1.4.* is, *a priori*, suitable for the encapsulation of DIMATE and MATE.

The aim of this study was to evaluate approaches for the preparation of ALDH1 inhibitor-loaded nanoparticles, and to test the *in vitro* biological activity of these formulations.

1.2. Aldehyde dehydrogenase inhibitors

The increased activity of enzymes that eliminate anti-tumor drugs or their metabolites is an important limiting factor in anticancer therapeutic protocols. Among these enzymes, aldehyde dehydrogenases 1 (ALDH1; ALDH1A1) and 3 (ALDH3; ALDH3A1) have been associated with drug resistance in some tumor cells [1]. In particular, their increased expression has been identified as a mechanism by which tumor cells may evade the cytotoxic effects exerted by the alkylating drug cyclophosphamide and its analogues, as well as that of anti-tumor drugs acting by free radical generation, for example doxorubicin [2]. It has also been observed that the activity of cytosolic ALDH3 in hepatoma cells increases in parallel with the degree of deviation and has been shown to be important in metabolizing cytostatic and cytotoxic aldehydes derived from lipid peroxidation [3]. These aldehydes, and in particular the most reactive product 4-hydroxynonenal, are known to cause a number of different effects including inhibition of cell proliferation and induction of apoptosis in both normal and tumor cells [4–8]. For this reason ALDH isoenzymes are important in regulating both drug resistance and cell proliferation. Their capacity to induce drug resistance has been confirmed by transfection studies in both tumor and normal cells. Resistance to oxazaphosphorines has been conferred to human MCF-7 breast cancer cells by transfection with ALDH3 cDNA, and to the murine L1210 hematopoietic cell line and human U937 cells by transfection with ALDH1 cDNA [9,10]. Moreover, overexpression of ALDH1 antisense RNA has been shown to induce resistance to 4-hydroperoxycyclophosphamide, the active metabolite of cyclophosphamide, in A459 lung cancer cells and in K562 leukemia cells [11].

On this basis, inhibitors of ALDH1 should, at least in theory, be capable of alleviating this chemoresistance. Quash et al. have designed and synthesized a novel group of inhibitors of ALDH1, 4-amino-4-methyl-pent-2-yn-1-al (ampal) and its analogues [12]. These compounds have not only proved to be good inhibitors of ALDH1, but also have demonstrated to inhibit cell growth of several tumor cells lines [1,12].

1.3. Nanoparticles as carriers of anticancer drugs

Nanoparticles prepared with biodegradable polymers (e.g. poly(alkylcyanoacrylate), poly(lactic acid) and poly[lactic-co-glycolic acid]) have been often investigated as delivery systems for anticancer agents [13–16]. In addition to being biocompatible, these colloidal carriers enable entrapment of compounds with different physicochemical characteristics and they can provide controlled release profiles of encapsulated drugs. Indeed, drugs incorporated into the nanoparticles are protected by the polymeric matrix from degradation during their transport within the body. In addition, nanoparticles can be administered by intravenous injection as well as by intramuscular and subcutaneous administration. If designed appropriately, in terms of size and surface characteristics, nanoparticles can be targeted to tumor tissues or cells. Once in contact with the cell, they can be endocytosed/phagocytosed which results in the cellular internalization of the encapsulated drug. At the tumor level, the accumulation mechanism of intravenously injected nanoparticles relies on a passive diffusion or convection across the leaky, hyperpermeable tumor vasculature. Examples of anticancer agents delivered from nanoparticulate systems include paclitaxel, doxorubicin and cystatin [13–16].

1.4. The novel emulsification-evaporation method

A novel emulsification-evaporation method, developed and patented by Quintanar et al. [17,18], involves the formation of an oil-in-water emulsion between a partially water-soluble solvent (e.g. methyl acetate, ethyl acetate, butanone) containing the polymer and the drug, and an aqueous phase containing a stabilizer (e.g. poly(vinyl alcohol) or poloxamer). After emulsification, the organic solvent is evaporated under vacuum, leading to polymer aggregation, which results in the formation of nanoparticles. Optionally, the organic solvent can be also extracted from the emulsion droplets by addition of a sufficient quantity of water to induce solvent diffusion into the external phase. Interestingly, this method allows the preparation of nanospheres as well as nanocapsules. In particular, the production of nanocapsules requires the incorporation of an oily substance, either the drug itself or an oily excipient (e.g. Miglyol® N812), in the organic phase [17–20].

Nanoparticles of a wide range of mean sizes, from 60 to 7000 nm, can be obtained by this novel technique of emulsification-evaporation. The mean size of nanoparticles is influenced by several factors: the internal/external volume ratio, the polymer content in the internal phase, the concentration of emulsifying agent in the external phase and the stirring rate. Another useful aspect of this technique is the flexibility with respect to formulation. Depending on the organic phase solvent, non-biodegradable (e.g. Eudragit®) as well as biodegradable polymers (e.g. poly(lactic acid), poly(lactic-co-glycolic acid) and poly[ε-caprolactone]) can be used for the preparation of nanoparticles [18–22].

Compared to other existing methods used for the production of nanoparticles, this process presents clear advantages, namely: a) high yields of nanoparticles in the final raw dispersion; b) the use of pharmaceutically acceptable organic solvents (e.g. ethyl acetate or butanone); c) the possibility of solvent recycling; d) simple implementation and ease of scaling-up; d) high reproducibility.

The selection of this novel method for preparing ALDH1 inhibitor-loaded nanoparticles was made in view of the following facts. Owing to the physical

state of the two ALDH1 inhibitors (Fig. 1), DIMATE (an oily liquid) and
MATE (a solid substance), they should be incorporated into nanocapsules and
nanospheres, respectively. At present, among the methods existing for the
manufacture of polymeric nanoparticles, only the above-mentioned
emulsification-evaporation method and the nanoprecipitation technique allow
the preparation of both types of nanoparticles. In particular, this novel
emulsification-evaporation method also allows significantly higher yields of
nanoparticles to be obtained relative to the nanoprecipitation technique.

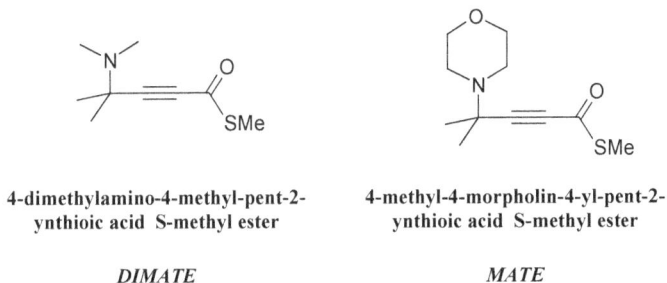

**4-dimethylamino-4-methyl-pent-2-
ynthioic acid S-methyl ester**

**4-methyl-4-morpholin-4-yl-pent-2-
ynthioic acid S-methyl ester**

DIMATE

MATE

Fig. 1. Molecular structure of aldehyde dehydrogenase inhibitors.

1.5. Aim of the study

The purpose of this study was to develop and characterize an optimal
formulation based on biodegradable nanoparticles (≤ 200 nm) containing
ALDH1 inhibitors which would be later evaluated in *in vitro* and *in vivo* studies.
Nanoparticles, in the form of nanocapsules or nanospheres, were prepared by the
emulsification-evaporation method using poly(lactic acid) as polymer.

2. MATERIALS AND METHODS

2.1. Materials

The novel ALDH1 inhibitors, DIMATE and MATE (Fig. 1), were provided by the research group of G. Quash (Laboratoire d'Immunochimie, Faculté de Médecine Lyon-Sud, France). Poly(D,L-lactic acid) (PLA) with a molecular weight of 12 000 Da (PLA 100 DL 2M®) was obtained from Medisorb Alkermes (Cincinnati, OH, USA). Epikuron® 170, (Lucas Meyer, Hambourg, Germany) and poloxamer 188 (Lutrol® F68, BASF, Ludwigshafen, Germany) were used as hydrophobic and hydrophilic surfactants, respectively. Miglyol® 812N (Hüls, Witten, Germany) was used as the oily phase for preparing blank nanocapsules. All other chemicals were of analytical grade.

2.2. Calculation of solubility parameter of DIMATE and MATE

A problem often encountered with novel compounds is the lack of information concerning their physicochemical properties. A complete preformulation study is sometimes difficult because the active molecule is only available in minute amounts. In our study, we were confronted with precisely this problem: the solubility properties of DIMATE and MATE were unknown. This information is crucial in the development of nanoparticles because selection of the manufacturing method is based on the solubilities of the drug and the polymer.

In order to overcome this problem, we decided to estimate theoretically the solubility behavior of both ALDH1 inhibitors. The Hildebrand solubility parameter (δ, $MPa^{1/2}$) was calculated using the group contribution theory based on the molar evaporation energy (U, kJ mol^{-1}) and the molar volume (V, cm^3 mol^{-1}). Equation 1 shows this relationship [23],

$$\delta = \left(\frac{-U}{V}\right)^{1/2} = \left(\frac{-\sum_z {}^z U}{\sum_z {}^z V}\right)^{1/2} \tag{1}$$

where z is each group that constitutes the molecule. It should be pointed out that other methods, which also allow the theoretical calculation of the solubility parameter (e.g. Hoftyzer-Van Krevelen or Hoy methods), were not used in this study because they did not present the data of all groups conforming the molecules of ALDH1 inhibitors; specifically, the contribution of the triple bound group (C $\equiv$ C).

2.3. Nanoparticle preparation and characterization

Nanoparticles were prepared according to the emulsification-evaporation method proposed by Quintanar and co-workers [21]. The standard procedure was modified in order to obtain sub-200 nm nanoparticles with a narrow particle size distribution. Briefly, ethyl acetate and water were mutually saturated for 5 min before use. Then, the organic phase was prepared by dissolving the polymer (50-300 mg), the hydrophobic surfactant (50 mg of Epikuron® 170 previously dissolved in 0.5 ml of ethanol), and one of the ALDH1 inhibitors (25 mg of either MATE or DIMATE) in ethyl acetate (25 ml). This organic phase was emulsified with the aqueous solution of poloxamer (40 ml at 1-5 %, w/v) by stirring first at 2000 rpm for 15 min with a four-bladed impeller (Eurostar digital stirrer, IKA, Staufen, Germany), then at 9500 rpm for 4 min with a homogenizer (Ultra-Turrax T25, IKA Labotechnik, Germany). The organic solvent was evaporated under reduced pressure in order to obtain the nanoparticle dispersion in a final volume of 10 ml. Finally, since the ALDH1 inhibitors were physically different, two type of polymeric nanoparticles were obtained. DIMATE, a hydrophobic liquid compound, was encapsulated into nanocapsules, while MATE, a hydrophobic solid substance, was incorporated in the polymer matrix of nanospheres.

Particle mean size and polydispersity index (P.I.) of nanoparticles were measured using a Zetasizer 3000HS® (Malvern Instruments Ltd., Worcestershire, U.K.). Three measurements on three different batches of each nanoparticle formulation were made to determine the mean particle diameter and standard deviation.

2.4. DIMATE and MATE content in the aqueous nanoparticle dispersion

The concentration of DIMATE in the aqueous dispersion of nanoparticles obtained after the evaporation stage was determined using an ultraviolet spectrophotometric method. A calibration curve for DIMATE was prepared in a system of solvents containing ethyl acetate:water (50:1, v:v) and the absorbance was measured at $\lambda_{max} = 263$ nm (Hewlett Packard 8453 Spectrophotometer, Germany). The molar absorptivity ($\varepsilon_{263\,nm}^{DIMATE}$) obtained from the calibration curve had a value of 5.88×10^{-3} L mol^{-1} cm^{-1} . The samples of the aqueous nanoparticle dispersion were dissolved in ethyl acetate and the DIMATE content was measured using the appropriate calibration curve. An ethyl acetate:water ration of 50:1 (v:v) was maintained for the samples prepared with the aqueous dispersion of nanoparticles.

A similar ultraviolet spectrophotometric method was developed in order to determine the MATE content in the dispersion of nanoparticles obtained after the solvent-evaporation step. The absorbance of the samples containing MATE was also measured at 263 nm. Here, $\varepsilon_{263\,nm}^{MATE}$ corresponded to 6.74×10^{-3} L mol^{-1} cm^{-1}.

2.5. Drug loading of MATE-loaded nanoparticles

Drug loading was indirectly determined by a combined ultrafiltration-centrifugation technique using a Microcon® centrifugal filter device (100 000 Da cutoff membrane, Millipore, U.S.A.). A sample of the nanosuspension was centrifuged and the free drug content in the filtrate was assayed by UV spectroscopy using the method previously described. MATE content in the nanoparticles was determined from the difference between the total amount of MATE used to prepare the nanoparticles and the amount of MATE present in the external aqueous phase.

2.6. Inhibitory effect of MATE-loaded nanoparticles on the cancer cell line DU145

An *in vitro* study was performed in order to determine the effect of the MATE-loaded-nanoparticles on the growth of cancer cells. The DU145 cells, from a brain human prostate carcinoma, were incubated with the following systems: an alcoholic solution of MATE, MATE-loaded-nanoparticles and blank nanoparticles. Both dispersions of nanoparticles were sterilized by filtration through a 0.22 μm membrane before use. The formulations containing MATE were evaluated at concentrations of 2, 5, 10, 15 and 20 μM. After 72 h, the viable cells were scored with hemocytometer through the exclusion of trypan blue.

3. RESULTS AND DISCUSSION

3.1. Solubility parameter of DIMATE and MATE

The solubility parameter calculated from the group contribution theory was of 20.66 and 22.42 $MPa^{1/2}$ for DIMATE and MATE, respectively. Ethyl acetate, which is used as solvent in the emulsification-evaporation method, has a δ value of 18.6 $MPa^{1/2}$. Since $\Delta\delta_{solvent-solute}$ should be small ($\approx$ 5) for good solubility [24], ethyl acetate can be considered as an appropriate solvent for both molecules.

3.2. Optimization of the emulsification-evaporation method

Two main process parameters, the polymer concentration in the organic phase and surfactant concentration in the aqueous phase, were varied from the standard procedure of the emulsification-evaporation method in order to obtain nanocapsules with a sub-200 nm size. Because the ALDH1 inhibitor DIMATE is a newly synthesized compound and its availability is limited, this optimization stage was carried out by substituting the DIMATE with Miglyol® 812N in the organic phase. Miglyol® 812N was selected because of its oily character that also allows the preparation of nanocapsules. Analysis of results was made considering that the mean size of nanoparticles is dependent on the size of the emulsion droplets formed during the emulsification step.

3.2.1. Influence of polymer concentration in the internal phase

As shown in Table I, the nanoparticle mean size increased with increasing polymer concentration in the organic phase. This phenomenon might be directly related to the viscosity of the internal phase which increased as the polymer concentration increased in the organic phase. Since a higher internal phase viscosity offers more resistance to dispersion in the external phase by the shear forces during emulsification, the emulsification efficiency diminished, thus leading to an increase in the mean size of the emulsion droplets. This was clearly observed at a surfactant concentration of 5 % (w/v), where the mean size of nanoparticles ranged from 128 to 187 nm when PLA concentrations varied from 0.25 to 1.50 % (w/v).

3.2.2. Influence of surfactant concentration in the aqueous phase

The effect of the stabilizer concentration (poloxamer) on the nanoparticle mean size was clearly evidenced at 1.5 % PLA in the organic phase (Table I). By increasing the surfactant concentration from 1 to 5 %, the nanoparticle mean size decreased from 240 to 187 nm. Likewise, lower polydispersity index values were obtained, which supposed that the droplet size distribution became more uniform. The surfactant contained in the continuous phase plays a key role during emulsification. The amphiphilic molecules first reduce the interfacial tension thus facilitating the incorporation of the dispersed phase into the continuous phase; and second, they stabilize the droplet during break-up thus reducing coalescence. Therefore, by increasing surfactant concentration in the continuous phase, more molecules of surfactant were available for covering the surface of droplets resulting in a reduction of the mean size of the emulsion droplet.

Table I. Influence of the poly(D,L-lactic acid) concentration in the organic phase and poloxamer concentration in the aqueous phase on the mean size of blank nanocapsules prepared by emulsification-evaporation

poly(D,L-lactic acid) in the organic phase (%, w/v)	Mean diameter [a] (nm) and polydispersity index [b] [P.I.] poloxamer in the aqueous phase (%, w/v)			
	1.0	2.0	3.0	5.0
0.25	------	------	------	128 [0.226]
0.38	------	------	------	132 [0.145]
0.75	190 [0.358]	204 [0.294]	167 [0.160]	155 [0.125]
1.50	~ 240 [c]	228 [0.151]	203 [0.107]	187 [0.122]

[a] Mean of three determinations from three different batches (Zetasizer 3000, Malvern Electronics, Malvern, England).
[b] Polydispersity index [P.I.] ranges from 0 to 1. A higher value indicates a less homogeneous size distribution of nanoparticles.
[c] Abundant presence of aggregates, which affected considerably the recovery of nanoparticles.

Once the emulsification-evaporation method for obtaining sub-200 nm nanoparticles with a homogeneous particle distribution was optimized, Miglyol® 812N was replaced by either DIMATE or MATE in order to produce drug-loaded nanocapsules and nanospheres, respectively.

3.3. Preparation and characterization of DIMATE-loaded nanocapsules

Since DIMATE-loaded nanocapsules will be tested *in vitro* and *in vivo*, the surfactant concentration in the dispersion of nanocapsules should be low. Therefore, based on the results in Table I, the sub-200 nm DIMATE-loaded nanoparticles were prepared using an aqueous phase containing 1 % (w/v) poloxamer and an organic phase containing 0.75 % (w/v) PLA.

For the first series of experiments, DIMATE-loaded nanoparticles obtained after the evaporation step showed acceptable characteristics in terms of mean size (133 nm) and polydispersity index (0.208). However, when the DIMATE content was determined in the aqueous nanoparticle dispersion, the results were disappointing. Only 13.6 % of the theoretical content of DIMATE was found in the nanosuspension, suggesting that DIMATE had either been degraded or lost during the preparation of nanoparticles.

Therefore, a second series of experiments was performed by monitoring the DIMATE content at each stage of the emulsification-evaporation method. The content of DIMATE in each sample was measured using the analytical method described in *Section 2.4*. In this second approach, the prepared nanoparticles had a mean size of 153 nm and a polydispersity index of 0.197. The DIMATE content determined at each stage of nanoparticle preparation is shown in Table

II. The results clearly show that the solvent-evaporation stage was the critical step during the preparation of nanoparticles. Only 19.4 % of DIMATE was found in the nanoparticle dispersion after evaporation. Because it was suspected that the solvent and the DIMATE could have been simultaneously evaporated, DIMATE was monitored in the rotavapor as well as in the recovered solvent. Surprisingly, 2.5 % of DIMATE was found on the walls of the rotavapor and the refrigerant while 48.9 % of the substance was determined in the recovered solvent.

Table II. DIMATE content determined at each stage of the preparation of
DIMATE-loaded nanoparticles using the emulsification-evaporation
technique

Fluid resulted from the different stages of nanoparticle preparation	DIMATE content (%, w/w) [a]
Organic phase	101.0
Emulsion prepared at 2000 rpm	100.7
Emulsion prepared at 9500 rpm	98.4
Suspension of nanoparticles after the evaporation step	19.4

[a] Content of DIMATE = 100 x (mg of MATE experimentally determined / theoretical content of DIMATE in mg).

These findings demonstrated that the low DIMATE content in the nanoparticle dispersion was mainly due to the loss of DIMATE during the evaporation step of nanoparticle preparation. Therefore, it was concluded that the emulsification-evaporation method was not convenient for preparing DIMATE-loaded nanocapsules.

3.4. Preparation and characterization of MATE-loaded nanospheres

MATE-loaded nanoparticles were prepared according to the procedure cited in *Section 2.3.* Nanoparticles showed a small mean size (128 nm) and a relatively homogeneous distribution (P.I. = 0.159). In contrast to the dispersion of DIMATE-loaded nanoparticles, for which a significant percentage of the active molecule was lost during nanoparticle preparation, 99.0 % of MATE was recovered in the aqueous nanoparticle dispersion. This demonstrated that the method of preparation of nanoparticles, mainly the solvent-evaporation step, did not affect the MATE content in the nanodispersion.

Because these results only evidenced the content of MATE in the whole nanodispersion, it was necessary to determine the percentage of MATE incorporated into the nanoparticles. Using the method cited in *Section 2.5.*, MATE loading in the nanospheres corresponded to 29.7 %. The low incorporation of the active molecule in the nanoparticles could be attributed to a several factors: i) MATE could have partitioned into the external aqueous phase during the emulsification process; the presence of poloxamer as well as the energy supply by the stirrer could have favored the partition phenomenon; ii) molecules of MATE could have diffused simultaneously with the solvent into the external phase of the dispersion during the evaporation step.

Since no evidence of the substance in a solid state was found in the nanoparticle dispersion, it was thus suspected that the presence of poloxamer could have induced the formation of a micellar solution of MATE. This hypothesis is supported by the fact that the critical micelle concentration (CMC) of poloxamer 188 is 0.09-0.1 % (w/v, 25°C) [25,26] and that poloxamer concentration of the nanoparticles dispersion after evaporation was 4.0 % (w/v). Therefore, under these conditions (40-fold the poloxamer CMC), the formation of a micelle solution is highly probable. Moreover, various authors have previously reported the utility of poloxamer 188 as a solubilizing vehicle for hydrophobic drugs [25–29]. In this context, it was thus determined that the emulsification-evaporation technique was not optimum for obtaining MATE-loaded nanoparticles.

3.5. Inhibitory effect of MATE-loaded nanoparticles on DU145 cells

The batch of MATE-loaded-nanoparticles prepared in *Section 3.4.* was evaluated *in vitro* in terms of its inhibitory capacity on the cancer cells. The study was performed according to the methodology described in *Section 2.6.* After a 72 h incubation, the MATE solution as well as MATE-loaded-nanoparticles had a similar effect on the growth of the DU145 cells (Fig. 2). Moreover, the IC_{50} values were 3.5 and 2.1 µM for the alcoholic solution and the loaded nanoparticles, respectively.

Although these results showed that the dispersion of nanoparticles did not markedly improve the inhibitory activity of MATE, it should be noted that MATE activity was preserved. This indicates that nanoparticle formulations are suitable for the administration of MATE and offer a means of delivery without the use of organic solvents. Obviously, this type of formulation would have more acceptability than the alcoholic solution for subsequent *in vivo* and clinical studies.

105

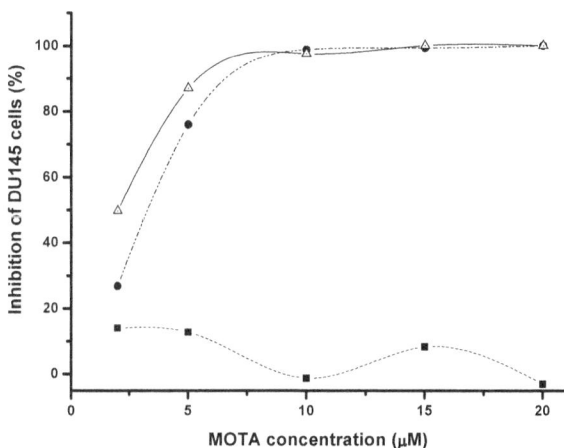

Fig. 2 Inhibitory effect of two different formulations of MATE on the DU145 cells: (●) alcoholic solution of MATE, (△) MATE-loaded nanoparticles and (■) drug-free nanoparticles.

4. CONCLUSIONS

The emulsification-evaporation method was employed for incorporating two ALDH1 inhibitors into polymeric nanoparticles. In general, this method was convenient neither for the production of DIMATE-loaded nanocapsules nor for MATE-loaded nanospheres.

In the case of DIMATE, significant amount of this molecule was lost during the preparation of nanoparticles. Therefore, it is proposed that other preparation methods for nanoparticles (e.g. salting-out, emulsification-diffusion and nanoprecipitation), which do not involve an evaporation process, should be tested for incorporating DIMATE into these colloidal carriers.

Further experiments should also be carried out in order to optimize MATE incorporation into nanospheres. First, a preformulation study of this active molecule, including the determination of MATE solubility in different solvents as well as the determination of its organic phase-aqueous phase partition coefficient, should be conducted. In addition, some strategies for improving the encapsulation of drugs into nanoparticles could be tested including incorporation of salts in the external phase [30,31], modification of the pH of the external phase [30–33], use of other solvents or mixtures of solvents in the organic phase [30,31] use of polymers with different molecular weight [32] and control of the evaporation rate of solvent during the preparation of nanoparticles [34]. Other techniques for the preparation of nanoparticles could be eventually tested.

With respect to the *in vitro* studies, it should be pointed out that although the nanoparticle dispersion contained only 29.7 % of MATE in the encapsulated form and the remainder free in the external aqueous phase, it showed a similar inhibitory activity to the alcoholic solution of MATE. Therefore, it is anticipated that by improving the incorporation of MATE into nanoparticles, its biological activity could be further enhanced.

Unfortunately, the present study had to be interrupted at this stage of the research because production of the ALDH1 inhibitors was suddenly discontinued.

Chapitre IV

ACKNOWLEDGEMENTS

The authors gratefully acknowledge G. Fournet from the Laboratoire de Chimie Organique, CPE-Lyon as well as J. Chantepie and G. Quash from the Laboratoire d'Immunochimie, Faculté de Médecine Lyon-Sud for their scientific collaboration. Likewise, authors are grateful to Dr. A. Naik for critically reviewing the manuscript.

REFERENCES

[1] R. A. Canuto, G. Muzio, R. A. Salvo, M. Maggiora, A. Trombetta, J. Chantepie, G. Fournet, U. Reichert, G. Quash, The effect of a novel irreversible inhibitor of aldehyde dehydrogenases 1 and 3 on tumour cell growth and death, Chem. Biol. Interact. 130-132 (2001) 209-218.

[2] N. E. Sladek, P. A. Dockham, M. O. Lee, Human and mouse hepatic aldehyde dehydrogenases important in the biotransformation of cyclophosphamide and the retinoids, Adv. Exp. Med. Biol. 284 (1991) 97-104.

[3] R. A. Canuto, M. Ferro, G. Muzio, A. M. Bassi, G. Leonarduzzi, M. Maggiora, D. Adamo, G. Poli, R. Lindahl, Role of aldehyde metabolizing enzymes in mediating effects of aldehyde products of lipid peroxidation in liver cells, Carcinogenesis 15 (1994) 1359-1364.

[4] R. A. Canuto, G. Muzio, M. Ferro, M. Maggiora, R. Federa, A. M. Bassi, R. Lindahl, M. U. Dianzani, Inhibition of Class-3 aldehyde dehydrogenase and cell growth by restored lipid peroxidation in hepatoma cell lines, Free Radic. Biol. Med. 26 (1999) 333-340.

[5] S. Pizzimenti, G. Barrera, M. U. Dianzani, S. Brusselbach, Inhibition of D1, D2, and a cyclin expression in HL-60 cells by the lipid peroxydation product 4-hydroxynonenal, Free Radic. Biol. Med. 26 (1999) 1578-1586.

108

Encapsulation de deux molécules possédant une activité anticancéreuse

[6] C. Cambiaggi, S. Dominici, M. Comporti, A. Pompella, Modulation of human T lymphocyte proliferation by 4-hydroxynonenal, the bioactive product of neutrophil-dependent lipid peroxidation, Life Sci. 61 (1997) 777-785.

[7] I. Kruman, A. J. Bruce-Keller, D. Bredesen, G. Waeg, M. P. Mattson, Evidence that 4-hydroxynonenal mediates oxidative stress-induced neuronal apoptosis, J. Neurosci. 17 (1997) 5089-5100.

[8] Y. Soh, K. S. Jeong, I. J. Lee, M. A. Bae, Y. C. Kim, B. J. Song, Selective activation of the c-Jun N-terminal protein kinase pathway during 4-hydroxynonenal-induced apoptosis of PC12 cells, Mol. Pharmacol. 58 (2000) 535-541.

[9] K. D. Bunting, R. Lindahl, A. J. Townsend, Oxazaphosphorine-specific resistance in human MCF-7 breast carcinoma cell lines expressing transfected rat class 3 aldehyde dehydrogenase, J. Biol. Chem. 269 (1994) 23197-23203.

[10] M. Magni, S. Shammah, R. Schiro, W. Mellado, R. Dalla-Favera, A. M. Gianni, Induction of cyclophosphamide-resistance by aldehyde-dehydrogenase gene transfer, Blood 87 (1996) 1097-1103.

[11] J. S. Moreb, C. Maccow, M. Schweder, J. Hecomovich, Expression of antisense RNA to aldehyde dehydrogenase class-1 sensitizes tumor cells to 4-hydroperoxycyclophosphamide in vitro, J. Pharmacol. Exp. Ther. 293 (2000) 390-396.

[12] G. Quash, G. Fournet, J. Chantepie, J. Gore, C. Ardiet, D. Ardail, Y. Michal, U. Reichert, Novel competitive irreversible inhibitors of aldehyde dehydrogenase (ALDH1): restoration of chemosensitivity of L1210 cells overexpressing ALDH1 and induction of apoptosis in BAF$_3$ cells overexpressing bcl$_2$, Biochem. Pharmacol. 64 (2002) 1279-1292.

[13] S. S. Feng, G. Huang, Effects of emulsifiers on the controlled release of paclitaxel (Taxol[®]) from nanospheres of biodegradable polymers, J. Control. Release 71 (2001) 53-69.

[14] I. Brigger, C. Dubernet, P. Couvreur, Nanoparticles in cancer therapy and diagnosis, Adv. Drug Del. Rev. 54 (2002) 631-651.

[15] S. S. Feng, S. Chien, Chemotherapeutic engineering: Application and further development of chemical engineering principles for chemotherapy of cancer and other diseases, Chem. Eng. Sci. 58 (2003) 4087-4114.

Chapitre IV

[16] M. Cegnar, J. Kos, J. Kristl, Cystatin incorporated in poly(lactide-*co*-glycolide) nanoparticles: development and fundamental studies on preservation of its activity, Eur. J. Pharm. Sci. 22 (2004) 357-364.

[17] D. Quintanar, H. Fessi, E. Doelker, E. Allémann. Procédé de préparation de nanocapsules de type vésiculaire, utilisables notamment comme vecteurs colloïdaux de principes actifs pharmaceutiques ou autres, France Patent 97 09 672, 1-20 (1997).

[18] D. Quintanar-Guerrero, E. Allémann, R. Gurny, H. Fessi, E. Doelker. Method for producing aqueous colloidal dispersions of nanoparticles, Patent WO 01/02087, 1-23 (2001).

[19] D. Quintanar-Guerrero, E. Allémann, E. Doelker, H. Fessi, Preparation and characterization of nanocapsules from preformed polymers by a new process based on emulsification-diffusion technique, Pharm. Res. 15 (1998) 1056-1062.

[20] S. Guinebretiere. Nanocapsules par emulsion-diffusion de solvant: obtention, caracterisation et mecanisme de formation, Thesis 200-2001, Claude Bernard University-Lyon 1, France, 1-245 (2001).

[21] D. Quintanar-Guerrero, E. Allémann, H. Fessi, E. Doelker, Pseudolatex preparation using a novel emulsion-diffusion process involving direct displacement of partially water-miscible solvents by distillation, Int. J. Pharm. 188 (1999) 155-164.

[22] C. A. Nguyen, Y. Konan-Kouakou, E. Allémann, E. Doelker, D. Quintanar-Guerrero, H. Fessi, R. Gurny, Novel method for the preparation of surfactant-free nanoparticles of methacrylic acid copolymers, In press AAPS Pharm. Sci. Tech. (2004).

[23] M. F. A. Barton, Homologous series and homomorphs. In: Handbook of Solubility Parameters and Other Cohesion Parameters, CRC Press, Boca Raton, Florida, U.S.A., 1st ed., 1985, pp. 61-89.

[24] D. W. Van Krevelen, Cohesive properties and solubility. In: Properties of Polymers, Elsevier, Amsterdam, Netherlands, 3rd ed., 1990, pp. 189-225.

[25] W. Saski, S. G. Shah, Availability of drugs in the presence of surface-active agents I : Critical micelle concentrations of some oxyethylene oxypropylene polymers, J. Pharm. Sci. 54 (1965) 71-74.

Encapsulation de deux molécules possédant une activité anticancéreuse

[26] M. F. Saettone, B. Giannaccini, G. Delmonte, V. Campigli, G. Tota, F. La Marca, Solubilization of tropicamide by poloxamers: physicochemical data and activity data in rabbits and humans, Int. J. Pharm. 43 (1988) 67-76.

[27] N. E. Hoffman, The relationship between uptake in vitro of oleic acid and micellar solubilization, Biochim. Biophys. Acta 196 (1970) 193-203.

[28] A. V. Kabanov, E. V. Batrakova, N. S. Melik-Nubarov, N. A. Fedoseev, T. Y. Dorodnich, V. Y. Alakhov, V. P. Chekhonin, I. R. Nazarova, V. A. Kabanov, A new class of drug carriers: micelles of poly(oxyethylene)-poly(oxypropylene) block copolymers as microcontainers for drug targeting from blood in brain, J. Control. Release 22 (1992) 141-157.

[29] M. A. Hammad, B. W. Muller, Solubility and stability of clonazepam in mixed micelles, Int. J. Pharm. 169 (1998) 55-64.

[30] I. Yamakawa, Y. Tsushima, R. Machida, S. Watanabe, Preparation of neurotensin analogue-containing poly(*d,l*-lactic acid) microspheres formed by oil-in-water solvent evaporation, J. Pharm. Sci. 81 (1992) 899-903.

[31] X. M. Deng, X. H. Li, M. L. Yuan, C. D. Xiong, Z. T. Huang, W. X. Jia, Y. H. Zhang, Optimization of preparative conditions for poly-D,L-lactide-polyethylene glycol microspheres with entrapped *Vibrio Cholera* antigens, J. Control. Release 58 (1999) 123-131.

[32] F. Gabor, B. Ertl, M. Wirth, R. Mallinger, Ketoprofen-poly(D,L-lactic-co-glycolic acid) microspheres: influence of manufacturing parameters and type of polymer on the release characteristics, J. Microencapsul. 16 (1999) 1-12.

[33] S. Galindo-Rodríguez, E. Allémann, E. Doelker, H. Fessi, Versatility of three techniques for preparing nanoparticles of different sizes and drug loadings, Submitted (2004).

[34] W. T. Chuang, Y. Y. Huang, L. Y. Tsai, Y. Z. Liu, Effects of solvent evaporation rate on the properties of protein-loaded PLLA and PDLLA microspheres fabricated by emulsion-solvent evaporation process, J. Microencapsul. 19 (2002) 463-471.

CHAPITRE V

NANOPARTICULES À BASE DE POLYMÈRES POUR L'ADMINISTRATION ORALE DES SUBSTANCES MÉDICAMENTEUSES ET DES VACCINS: ÉTUDES *in vivo*

POLYMERIC NANOPARTICLES FOR ORAL DELIVERY OF DRUGS AND VACCINES: CRITICAL EVALUATION OF *in vivo* STUDIES

S. Galindo-Rodríguez [1,2,3], *E. Allémann* [2,4], *H. Fessi* [3] *and E. Doelker* [2]

[1] Pharmapeptides, Geneva-Lyon Interuniversity Center, 74166 Archamps, France.

[2] School of Pharmacy, University of Geneva, 1211 Geneva 4, Switzerland.

[3] UMR-CNRS 5007, Faculty of Pharmacy, Claude Bernard University Lyon I, 69373 Lyon, France.

[4] Bracco Research SA, Plan-les-Ouates, 1228 Geneva, Switzerland.

Submitted to Critical Reviews in Therapeutic Drug Carriers Systems

Abstract

Oral drug delivery is the preferred route of administration of drugs. Because of their versatility and wide range properties, nanoparticles have been often investigated for delivery a wide number of drugs by this route. This paper first examines the physicochemical, pharmaceutical and technological aspects that make of nanoparticles a potential oral delivery system of drugs and active biomolecules. Next, upon consideration of *in vivo* studies, the pharmacokinetic, pharmacological and therapeutic aspects of nanoparticles orally administered are described. Special emphasis is made on improvement of oral bioavailability of drugs incorporated into nanoparticles. Two main mechanisms involved in enhancing drug absorption – the protection of drug by nanoparticles against harsh conditions in the gut as well as the prolongation of gastrointestinal transit of nanoparticles by using bioadhesive polymers – are analyzed. Furthermore, nanoparticle uptake by intestinal cells and oral vaccination by these colloidal carriers are also covered. In this context, the immune responses elicited as well as the protection against pathogens induced by antigen-loaded nanoparticles administered by oral route are presented. Finally, main limitations and perspectives of these colloidal carriers as oral drug delivery systems are discussed.

Chapitre V

Keywords : nanoparticles; colloidal carriers; oral drug delivery; bioadhesive nanoparticles; *in vivo* studies; nanoparticle uptake; oral vaccination; DNA vaccines; peptide encapsulation; oral bioavailability;

CONTENTS

1. Introduction

Oral drug delivery is the most preferred route for administrating drugs due to its non-invasive nature. In fact, the oral route presents a series of attractive advantages such as the avoidance of pain and discomfort associated with injections and the elimination of possible infections caused by the use of needles. Moreover, oral formulations are less expensive to produce, because they do not need to be manufactured under sterile conditions. However, numerous drugs remain poorly available when administered by this route. This is mainly due to: i) low mucosal permeability for the drug; ii) drug absorption restricted to a region of the gastrointestinal (GI) tract;   iii) low or very low solubility of the compound, which results in a slow dissolution in the mucosal fluids and elimination of a large fraction of the drug from the GI tract prior to absorption; and   iv) lack of stability in the GI environment, resulting in a degradation of the compound prior to its absorption (e.g. peptides, proteins). Among other approaches, it has been proposed to associate drugs with colloidal carriers such as polymeric nanoparticles to circumvent these problems.

2. Polymeric nanoparticles

2.1. Definition

Polymeric nanoparticles are solid colloid carriers ranging in size from 10 to 1000 nm.   They consist of macromolecular materials in which the active principle (drug or biologically active material) is dissolved, entrapped, encapsulated and/or to which the active principle is adsorbed or coupled to the surface. Structurally, two types of nanoparticles can be identified: nanospheres and nanocapsules. Nanospheres are monolithic particles possessing a porous or solid polymer matrix, while nanocapsules consist of a polymeric membrane surrounding a solid or liquid drug reservoir.

2.2. Significance of physicochemical characteristics of nanoparticles

Several reasons make of nanoparticles promising systems for oral drug delivery. From a physicochemical point of view, the favorable characteristics of nanoparticles such as sub-micron size, large specific surface area, multiparticulate character and variable polymer composition confer to these carriers a singular behavior in the GI tract.

Due to their sub-micron size, nanoparticles can either adhere directly to the mucus network or penetrate in the mucus layer and bind to the underlying epithelium. In this context, two events are possible: i) nanoparticles entrapped into the villi network may be retained in the intestine for longer times than larger oral dosage forms (e.g. capsules or tablets) [1]; or ii) nanoparticles might be internalized by the intestinal cells which allows an efficient delivery of therapeutic agents to target sites in the body. This implies that nanoparticles can be used either for enhancing the local delivery of drugs (e.g. for the treatments of pathogens localized in tissues of the GI) [2] or for promoting the oral absorption of active substances which have a systemic action [3-5].

With respect to the great specific surface area of nanoparticles, this can offer the following advantages: i) an extended number of drug molecules can be adsorbed and thus carried by the nanoparticles; ii) a large surface area is available for partitioning the encapsulated drug which can result in increased rates of dissolution; iii) an intimate and close contact can be established between the dosage form and the intestinal mucosa; and finally, iv) the surface modification of the particle can be tailored by adsorption or chemical grafting of certain molecules (e.g. poly(ethylene glycol) (PEG), poloxamers, poloxamines and bioactive molecules such as lectins and invasins) on the particle surface. The multiparticulate character and variable polymer composition of nanoparticles will be later discussed.

117

Chapitre V

2.3. *Pharmaceutical and formulation aspects of nanoparticles*

2.3.1. *Drug incorporation into nanoparticles*

Polymeric nanoparticles are also of interest from the pharmaceutical viewpoint. Depending on the method used for nanoparticle preparation, hydrophilic as well as hydrophobic drugs can be associated to these colloidal carriers. In fact, the active substance can be found encapsulated into the nanoparticle core (oily compounds or drugs soluble in an oil) [6], adsorbed onto the nanoparticle surface (mainly hydrophilic drugs) [7] or dispersed in the polymer matrix (hydrophobic and hydrophilic drugs) [8]. Moreover, certain compounds can be covalently bound to polymeric matrix [9]. However, for the latter option, it is necessary to ascertain that the biological activity of the drug is kept [10].

2.3.2. *Importance of the polymer composition of the nanoparticles*

Several polymeric materials can be used for preparing nanoparticles which enable the modulation of physicochemical characteristics (e.g. hydrophobicity, zeta potential), drug release properties (e.g. extended, triggered) and biological behavior of nanoparticles (e.g. biorecognition, bioadhesion, cellular uptake). Polymeric materials used for the formulation of these colloidal carriers include synthetic polymers such as poly(lactide acid), poly(lactide-*co*-glycolide), poly(ε-caprolactone), poly(methylmethacrylates), and poly(alkylcyanoacrylates) or natural polymers such as albumin, gelatin, alginate, collagen and chitosan. While natural polymers generally provide a relatively short duration of drug release, synthetic polymers enable to extend the release of the encapsulated therapeutic agents over periods of days to several weeks. Depending on the polymer nature, the entrapped drug can be released by diffusion from the polymer matrix as well as by degradation or dissolution of the polymer matrix [11]. For the case of biodegradable polymers, e.g. poly(lactide-*co*-glycolide), drug release from the nanoparticles can be controlled by the polymer degradation rate, which in turn is determined by the composition, molecular weight and crystallinity degree of the polymer [12]. It has also shown that the release rate of therapeutic agents from alginate nanoparticles can be controlled depending on their crosslinking degree [13]. Several *in vivo* studies have reported that nanoparticles can not only provide extended release of encapsulated drugs but also improve the plasma profile of the absorbed drug [14-16].

On the other hand, nanoparticles designed with mucoadhesive polymers can offer additional advantages when they are orally administered. In the case of drugs having a narrow absorption window in the intestine, bioadhesive nanoparticles might not only localize the drug carrier in a specific site but also extent its residence there. Because this leads to the creation of a high drug concentration gradient in the localized zone of the GI tract, an efficient absorption and thus an enhanced bioavailability of the drugs is achieved [17]. In addition, nanoparticles prepared with bioadhesive and bioerodible polymers undergo selective uptake by the M cells of Peyer patches in GI mucosa. Interestingly, this uptake mechanism has been utilized for the delivery of protein and peptide drugs, antigens for vaccination and plasmid DNA for gene therapy. Finally, by using methacrylic acid copolymers, it is possible to prepare pH sensitive nanoparticles which can potentially deliver the drug in selected regions of the GI tract [18-20].

2.3.3. Comparison of nanoparticles with other oral dosage forms

Nanoparticles offer several advantages over other oral dosage forms. When compared to single-unit preparations (e.g. tablets and capsules), multiparticulate systems, such as nanoparticules, distribute more uniformly in the GI tract. This results in a more uniform drug absorption and a reduced risk of local irritation [21,22]. Now, comparing with other multiparticulate carriers (e.g. microspheres or pellets), the smaller size of nanoparticles is considered a key parameter. Whereas nanoparticles are assumed to penetrate the mucus layer and to reach the apical membrane of the ephitelium cells, microparticles larger than 10 μm in diameter are excluded by the viscous gel layer of mucus [23]. Moreover, nanoparticles are taken up by intestinal cells better than microparticles [24]. It was found that the number of nanoparticles which cross the intestinal epithelium is greater than the number of microspheres. The uptake exclusion was evident for particles larger than 4 μm.

Nanoparticles have also evidenced advantages over other colloidal carriers. Nanoparticles have distinctly shown to be more stable than liposomes in biological fluids [25]. Various studies clearly demonstrated that liposomes were not likely to be stable in the gastrointestinal tract, particularly in the presence of bile salts [26,27]. It is obvious that drugs entrapped in liposomes are released if the physical structure of the carrier is disrupted. Moreover, endocytosis of intact liposomes by the intestinal cells, if it occurs at all, is a rare event [27], thus discarding the potential application of these colloidal carriers for oral use to improve the GI passage of poorly absorbed potent drugs.

2.3.4. Oral dosage form based on polymeric nanoparticles

Considering the practical aspect of their oral administration, nanoparticles can be kept in suspension or converted into a powder, usually by lyophilization or spray drying. For the first case, nanoparticle suspension might be administered as such. Alternatively, the aqueous dispersion of nanoparticles can be directly incorporated into the solid dosage forms, for example by granulation with other excipients to form granules or possibly tablets, or through layering of the dispersion onto pellets in a fluidized bed [28]. Likewise, nanoparticles can be entrapped in beads which might be administered as prepared or be filled into capsules [21]. In all cases, the polymeric nanoparticles should be discharged completely with their original properties (e.g. particle size distribution) in order to maintain the advantages of colloidal carriers for oral drug delivery. In the second case, lyophilized nanoparticles also offer alternatives for preparing oral formulations. Due to their free dispersion in water [29], lyophilized nanoparticles could be formulated as powders for extemporaneous preparations. Vehicles used for preparing the oral suspensions of nanoparticles include aqueous solutions, oils [30], mucoadhesive gels [14,15] and microemulsions [31]. In addition, after mixing with the compatible excipients, the dried powder of nanoparticles can also be filled into hard gelatin capsules. On the other hand, the compression of granules containing nanoparticles for preparing tablets is an unit operation not recommended mainly because, under high pressure, the integrity of particles can be drastically affected. Even, the possible fusion of polymeric nanoparticles during compression could result in a non-disintegrating matrix with the loss of their character of a multiparticulate dosage form.

2.4. Technological aspects of nanoparticles: manufacturing methods and scaling-up

Technologically, a large number of methods exist for the manufacture of particles with sub-micron sizes, allowing extensive modulation of their structure, composition, and physicochemical properties. The choice of the manufacturing method essentially depends on the raw material intended to be used and on the solubility characteristics of the active compound to be associated to the nanoparticles. Information about this topic can be read in recent reviews [32-34]. Interestingly, several preparation methods of polymeric nanoparticles have been scaled up which shows that the production of these colloidal carriers at large scale is highly feasible [35-38].

3. *In vivo* studies using nanoparticles for oral delivery of drugs

The use of nanoparticles as oral drug delivery systems has been proposed to improve the bioavailability of drugs with poor absorption characteristics [39,40], to treat local infections in the GI tract [2], reduce the irritating effects of some drugs (e.g. indomethacin, diclofenac) on the GI mucosa [41-43] and protect labile compounds (e.g. peptides, proteins and nucleic acids) from degradation in the GI tract [5,31,44-46].

3.1. Delivery of drugs for treatment of local infections in the gastrointestinal tract

Nanoparticulate systems have been proposed for improving the local treatment of pathogens infecting the intestinal tissues. The presence of human immunodeficiency virus (HIV) in the intestinal tract of the HIV-positive patients has been associated to pathologic effects such as chronic diarrhea [47]. So, a formulation of poly(isohexylcyanoacrylate) nanospheres containing 3'-azido 3'-deoxythymidine (AZT) has been developed to concentrate the drug in the intestinal epithelium and associated immunocompetent cells, which are known to be one of the major reservoirs of the virus [2]. Ninety minutes after intragastric administration to rats, nanospheres were able to concentrate at least 5.9 times AZT in the GI tract when compared to a control water solution. In particular, concentrations in the stomach and intestine were higher than in the caecum and colon. It was also noted that nanospheres concentrated efficiently AZT in Peyer's patches, specifically 4-fold greater than the solution. The ability of nanoparticles for increasing the drug concentration in these regions of the GI tract was attributed to their immobilization by the mucus. Because such immobilization increased the contact time of the carrier with the tissues, authors suggested that nanoparticles would act as a regular deposit of the drug along the intestine allowing the release of drug for a prolonged time. So, these findings supported the view that nanoparticles may represent a promising carrier to treat locally the GI reservoir of HIV [2].

3.2. Protection against the gastrointestinal irritating ulcerative effects of drugs

Side effects of drugs into the GI tract, such as irritation and mucosal damage, can be diminished by using polymeric nanoparticles. Non-steroidal anti-inflammatory drugs have been candidates for evaluating this beneficial effect of nanoparticles. The GI lesions induced by these drugs depend on two different mechanisms: a local action exerted by a direct contact with the GI mucosa and a generalized systemic action taking place following absorption. Guterres et al. [43] determined that the irritancy of diclofenac and indomethacin was drastically diminished in all sections of the GI tract when the drugs were incorporated into nanocapsules. This was explained by two facts, first nanocapsules limited the direct contact of the free drugs with the mucosa and second, nanocapsules released slowly the drugs thus avoiding their high local concentrations. Concerning the biological activity, it had been previously demonstrated that encapsulation of indometacin affected significantly neither its bioavailability nor its pharmacological activity in rats [42,48]. In particular, the relative bioavailability of indometacin-loaded nanoparticles, calculated from the ratio of AUC of nanocapsules / AUC of aqueous solution, had a value of 0.84 [48].

3.3. Reduction in dosing frequency and systemic toxic effects of drugs

Nanoparticles have been also proposed for reducing the dosing frequency of drugs. Pandey et. al. [49] reported the formulation of three frontline antitubercular drugs (i.e. rifampicin, isoniazid and pyrazinamide) encapsulated in poly(D,L-lactide-co-glycolide) nanoparticles. Following the oral administration of drug-loaded nanoparticles to mice, the drugs were detected in the circulation for 6 days (rifampicin) and 9 days (isoniazid and pyrazinamide), whereas therapeutic concentrations in the tissues were maintained for 9 to 11 days. This is in contrast to free drugs which were cleared from the plasma within 12 to 24 h of oral administration. Further, after oral administration of drug-loaded nanoparticles to *Mycobacterium tuberculosis*-infected mice every 10 days, no tubercle bacilli were detected in the tissues after 5 oral doses of treatment. From drug accumulation studies as well as hepatotoxicity analysis, it was shown that nanoparticles can drastically reduce drug toxic effects. The reduced toxicity was probably due to the slower and more controlled release of drugs from nanoparticles than free drugs. It was also proposed that the bioadhesion of nanoparticles to the intestinal mucosa might contribute to this effect. It was also noted that the dosing frequency of the treatment were significantly reduced from 46 doses (for free drugs daily) to 5 doses (drug-loaded nanoparticles every 10 days). In general, the formulation of nanoparticles bears important implications for tuberculosis therapy because reduction in dosing frequency would certainly enhance the patient compliance and, hence, better management of the disease [49].

Encapsulation of darodipine, a dihydropyridine calcium entry blocker, is another example in which formulations of nanoparticles could aid to diminish the risk of adverse effects. Darodipine, a potent hypotensive agent, may cause a rapid and pronounced fall in blood pressure to levels at which iatrogenic cerebral ischemia could occur. So, in order to prevent this adverse effect, darodipine was formulated into poly(isobutylcyanoarcylate) nanocapsules [4]. After oral administration to hypertensive rats, the relative bioavailability of the darodipine-loaded nanocapsules was 1.05 which indicated that the encapsulation of darodipine did not diminish its intestinal absorption. In addition, when compared to a darodipine-PEG formulation, nanocapsules presented a less pronounced initial hypotensive effect. This attenuation in the pharmacological effect of darodipine suggests that its encapsulation may diminish the risk of the cerebral ischemia induced by a rapid fall in blood pressure [4].

3.4. Use of nanoparticles for prophylactic therapies

Nanoparticles orally administered have also shown to be useful in prophylactic therapies. Interesting results were obtained with insulin [50]. Now that subjects at risk for diabetes can be identified, a major goal is to reduce the incidence of diabetes by disease-specific nontoxic therapies, including prophylactic insulin therapy. Since several studies have reported the prophylactic effect of early insulin injections on rodents, it was thus postulated that an oral dosage form of insulin could be also convenient for this end [50]. Using the nonobese diabetic mouse model, which mimics human type 1 diabetes, insulin-loaded nanocapsules led to a reduction in the incidence of diabetes, a delay of the onset of the disease and a diminution in the severity of the lymphocytic inflammation of endogenous islets. The prophylactic effect remained even 60 days after that the treatment was stopped. In general, this form of prophylactic insulin administration would be more comfortable and less constraining than parenteral administration.

3.5. Enhancement of oral bioavailability of drugs

A number of drugs has been incorporated into nanoparticles with the aim of improving their oral bioavailability and thus their pharmacological effect. Basically, these colloidal carriers enhance the oral absorption of drugs by means of two main mechanisms: they protect the encapsulated drug against the harsh conditions of the stomach and intestines, and also they increase the residence time of the drug during its transit through the GI tract. In addition, the vehicle used for oral administration of nanoparticles has also an influence on the oral absorption of the encapsulated drug.

3.5.1. Protection of drugs of the gastrointestinal environment

One way to enhance oral absorption of a drug is to improve its stability in the GI tract. Considering that a drug incorporated into the nanoparticles is surrounded by a polymer network, it is expected that this polymeric barrier protects the drug from the environment of the GI. A study carried out by Damgé et al. [51] illustrates this protective effect of the polymeric nanoparticles. The authors investigated the *in vitro* stability of insulin, associated to poly(isobutylcyanoacrylate) nanospheres or not, in presence of digestive enzymes. Free insulin was markedly degraded in presence of the pepsin, trypsin and chymotrypsin. Only 11 % of the initial amount of insulin remained undegraded after incubation with pepsin and trypsin and 23 % after incubation with chymotrypsin. In contrast, 75 to 85 % of the initial amount of insulin associated to nanospheres was recovered after incubation of nanospheres with pepsin and 80 to 95 % after incubation with chymotrypsin. In the presence of trypsin, insulin incorporated in nanospheres was well preserved (83 %) only when nanospheres were dispersed in an oily medium. It was also determined that, after a single peroral administration to rats, the hypoglycemic effect of insulin loaded into nanospheres was improved when compared to free insulin. Other studies performed by the same research group revealed that not only nanospheres but also nanocapsules can protect insulin against proteolytic enzymes of the GI tract [44].

In an interesting study, Low and Temple [5] observed that, when incorporated into nanocapsules, both insulin and calcitonin were significantly more resistant to protease degradation than free peptides in solution. Further, considering that the small intestinal lumen does not contain proteases alone, but also bile, a

127

second approach was made by incorporating a bile extract. Although still significant, the protection offered by nanoencapsulation was reduced by the introduction of bile extract. It seemed that the surfactant bile acids aided in the disruption of the oily core of the nanocapsules and allowed lipases to hydrolyze the triglyceride oil. Subsequently, these *in vitro* experiments were correlated with plasma pharmacokinetic profiles obtained after administration of nanocapsule formulations in the duodenum of rats. Higher plasma concentrations of the peptides were detected in the later times, which reflected the protective effect of nanocapsules. However, it was determined that the nanocapsule formulations gave no significant overall enhancement of peptide bioavailability.

Watnasirichaikul et al. [31] carried out *in vitro* release studies and determined that poly(isobutylcyanoacrylate) nanocapsules could suppress insulin release under acidic conditions (pH=1.2) and hence may protect the entrapped protein during its transit through the stomach. The biological activity of the insulin contained in the nanocapsules was confirmed by the pharmacodynamic response obtained after the oral administration of this formulation. Likewise, these findings were in agreement with a previous study of Scherer and co-workers [52] who, from an *in vitro* study simulating the conditions of the GI tract, also demonstrated that poly(butylcyanoacrylate) nanoparticles were stable enough to protect drugs against degradation in the GI tract.

It seems that the protective effect of nanoparticles depends on their polymeric composition. The effect of nanoparticles on the stability of salmon calcitonin (sCT) in the presence of digestive enzymes was investigated *in vitro* and correlated with the biological activity of the peptide [45,53,54]. Structurally, the polystyrene-based nanoparticles used in this study presented different hydrophilic polymeric chains on their surfaces. So, it was observed that the stabilization of sCT was affected by the structure of the hydrophilic polymeric chains. Poly(vinylamine) (PVAm) nanoparticles protected sCT against degradation by pepsin and trypsin. Poly(N-isopropylacrylamide) (PNIPAAm) nanoparticles inhibited completely sCT degradation by pepsin. Likewise, no degradation of sCT by trypsin occurred at all when poly(methacrylic acid) (PMAA) was the polymer. The poly(N-vinylacetamide) (PNVA) nanoparticles had a very limited stabilization for sCT [45]. Regarding *in vivo* study, sCT absorption was increased significantly by nanoparticles formed of PNIPAAm followed by those constituted of PVAm and PMAA. However, there was no absorption enhancement of sCT when PNVA was used as polymer [53]. The correlation of both studies suggested that the absorption enhancement of sCT in the GI tract could be ascribed in part to the stabilizing effect of nanoparticles on the enzymatic degradation of sCT [54].

Tobio et al. [46,55] determined that a PEG coating around poly(lactic acid) (PLA-PEG) nanoparticles improves the stability of these colloids in the GI fluids and their ability to transport ^{125}I-radiolabeled tetanus toxoid through the intestinal mucosa. The enzyme mediated aggregation of PLA nanoparticles was evaluated considering their agglomeration followed by their precipitation in simulated GI fluids. After 4 h incubation in gastric fluid, the percentage of non-aggregated nanoparticles was 90 % for PLA-PEG nanoparticles whereas only 10 % for PLA nanoparticles. Indeed, 57 % of the PLA-PEG nanoparticles remained stable whereas only 34 % of PLA nanoparticles maintained their integrity. With regard to polymer integrity, PLA forming the nanoparticles was found to be only slightly degraded which corresponded to 9 % for PLA nanoparticles and 4 % for PLA-PEG nanoparticles. It was also observed that the encapsulated tetanus toxoid remained mostly associated to the nanoparticles upon incubation in the digestive fluids for up to 4 h. These findings were confirmed with the *in vivo* studies showing that, after oral administration to rats, the level of encapsulated radioactive antigen in the blood stream was 5-fold higher for PLA-PEG nanoparticles than for those of PLA. The lymph nodes and stomach also showed significantly higher levels of antigen for PLA-PEG nanoparticles. It was probable that the stabilizing effect of the PEG-coating in the GI tract was due to the recognized protein repellent effect of PEG-coated surfaces which could reduce the degradation of PLA by the pancreatic lipase.

3.5.2. Prolongation of the gastrointestinal transit of drugs by the use of bioadhesive nanoparticles

Another strategy used for improving the bioavailability of poorly absorbed drugs is based on developing nanoparticulate carriers with bioadhesive properties [56,57]. One of the problems of peroral drug delivery is the limited and variable GI transit time of the dosage forms. When administered orally, nanoparticles follow at least three different pathways: i) direct transit and faecal elimination, ii) bioadhesion, or iii) uptake by the intestinal cells [56,58]. Particles undergoing no interactions with the mucosa and direct transit through the GI tract represent generally an important fraction of the dose administered. Kreuter et al. [1] observed that, after peroral administration of poly(hexyl-[3-^{14}C]-cyanoacrylate) nanoparticles to mice, particles were retained only at a level of 30-40 % for 8 h and about 5 % after 24 h. For this reason, a further prolongation of the GI transit time of the nanoparticles is desirable. One of the possibilities to achieve this goal is the development of bioadhesive nanoparticles which, by interaction with a biological subtract (e.g. mucus or intestinal cells), can be immobilized in the GI tract. In addition, nanoparticles having bioadhesive properties could offer other advantages: i) a localization at a given target site, e.g. the upper or lower GI tract; ii) an increased contact with the intestinal mucosa, resulting in a steep concentration gradient favoring drug absorption; and iii) a direct contact with intestinal cells which is the preliminary step for nanoparticle uptake [56,59].

Basically, two kind of bioadhesive interactions can be identified between the nanoparticles and the intestinal surfaces: i) non-specific interactions which are driven by the physicochemical properties of the particles (e.g. mean size, polymeric composition, hydrophobic-hydrophilic character) and the intestinal surfaces, and ii) specific interactions in which a ligand (e.g. lectins, adhesins) attached to the particle is used for the recognition and attachment to a specific site at the mucosal surface. Both type of interactions have been closely related to the functionality of bioadhesive nanoparticles in the GI tract. They are described in the following sections.

Nonspecific bioadhesive particulate systems
When nanoparticulate systems are orally administered, they first enter in contact with the GI fluids, and then with the mucin layer located on the mucosal membranes of the GI tract. Polymers forming nanoparticles, either of natural or synthetic origin, with the ability for adhering to that mucin layer are commonly named "mucoadhesives". Different types of bonding, such as van der Waals forces and hydrogen bonding, contribute to develop the mucoadhesive-mucin interaction. Because these types of interactions do not allow a selective adhesion of the polymer in the GI tract, mucoadhesive polymers are often

recognized as non-specific bioadhesive systems. So, it has been established that the intensity of interaction of non-specific bioadhesive nanoparticles with the GI mucosal membranes mainly depend on the intrinsic properties of the nanoparticles (e.g. size, density, surface properties) and the physicochemical characteristics of the polymer (e.g. hydrophobicity, charge, molecular weight, crosslinking degree) forming them.

Durrer et al. [60] evidenced that the adsorption behavior of nanoparticles on the intestinal mucosa strongly depends on the particle size. Adsorption isotherms of poly(styrene) latexes on rat intestinal mucosa were obtained using an *ex vivo* model and analyzed according to different adsorption models. Small latexes, sized between 200 and 670 nm, presented the characteristic isotherm shape of adsorbates which penetrate into the porous adsorbent. In contrast, particles larger than 2000 nm showed a Langmuir isotherm which corresponds to a monolayer of adsorbed particles on the surface of mucosa (Figure 1). In particular, the hypothesis of a diffusion of small particles into the mucous layer was further supported by a confocal microscopy study performed by Scherer and co-workers [17]. They showed that 200 nm particles penetrated at least 60 μm deep into the mucus layer of rat intestine mucosal fragments.

Lamprecht et coll. [23] investigated the size-dependent bioadhesion of particulate carriers to the inflamed colonic mucosa of rats. The highest binding to the inflamed colon (tissue and mucus) was found for 0.1 μm particles (14.5 % of administered particle mass). Particles with 1.0 μm in size showed a lower binding (9.1 %) while for 10 μm particles only fair deposition was observed (5.2 %). In addition, it was noted that a high amount of the particles were associated to the thicker mucus layer rather than attached or internalized by intestinal cells.

The percentage of particles only associated to the mucus was also size-dependent and corresponded to 61.4, 68.9 and 86.6% for particles of 0.1, 1.0 and 10 μm, respectively. Based on this results, authors also determined the residence time of 0.1 μm particles in the inflamed colon. Three days after oral administration of nanoparticles, a wash-out procedure was daily repeated during 6 days in order to recover the fraction of particles unassociated to the colon. It was found that 14.5 and 9.1 % of the initial dose of particles were retained in the colon after 1 and 2 days, respectively. A further decrease was observed after 4 and 6 days (3.4 and 1.9 %, respectively).

The mucoadhesion as well as the GI transit time of nanoparticles can also be influenced by their surface properties. Using a perfused rat ileum test system, Pimienta et al. [61] determined that coating poly(isohexylcyanoacrylate) nanospheres with poloxamer allows greater mucoadhesion, as compared with poloxamine-coated nanospheres. Kawashima et al. observed [62] that the mucoadhesion properties of poly(lactide-*co*-glycolide) nanospheres coated with various grades of chitosan varies as function of the molecular weight of chitosan. (MW 1500, 20'000, 50'000). The mucoadhesion of polymer increased parallel to its molecular weight. Authors proposed that the mucoadhesion properties of chitosan-coated particles may be due to the electrostatic attraction between the negatively charged mucus layer of the intestine and the positively charged polymer, as well as physical entanglements between the chitosan molecule and mucus components, depending on the molecular weight of chitosan.

The crosslinking degree of polymers used for preparing nanoparticles is another important factor associated to the mucoadhesion of nanoparticles in the GI tract.

133

Formulations of poly(methylvinylether-*co*-maleic anhydride) (PVM/MA) nanoparticles with different crosslinking degrees were administered by the oral route to fasted rats. It was determined that the gastric and intestinal emptying rates increased by increasing the extent of crosslinking of nanoparticles.

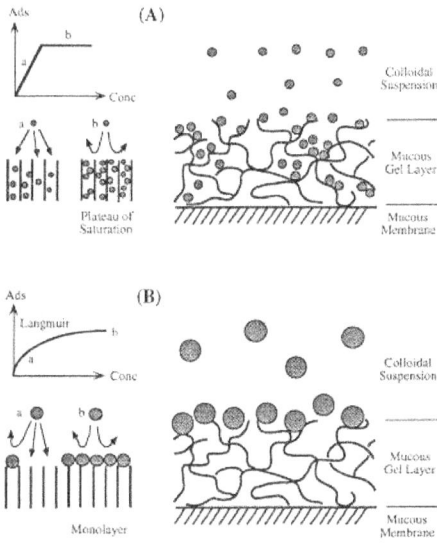

Figure 1. Adsorption isotherms and corresponding adsorption models. Adapted from reference [58].

It was also noted that the capacity to develop adhesive interactions and the intensity of the adhesive phenomenon were higher for conventional nanoparticles than for crosslinked carriers. It seemed that crosslinking of PVM/MA nanoparticles would block the adhesive active groups (e.g. carboxylic groups) at the nanoparticle surface thus decreasing their capacity to establish adhesive interactions with the mucosa [63]. Similar results were obtained for gliadin nanoparticles, which displayed a higher capacity to interact with the mucosa than nanoparticles crosslinked with glutaraldehyde [16].

Relationship between the mucoadhesive properties of nanoparticles and the improvement in the oral absorption of encapsulated drugs

Sakuma et al. investigated [54,64] the relationship among mucoadhesion of polystyrene nanoparticles having surface hydrophilic chains, their intestinal transit and the enhancement of *in vivo* sCT absorption in rats. The GI transit rates of nanoparticles having surface PNIPAAm, PVAm and PMAA chains, which improve sCT absorption, were lower than that of nanoparticles covered by PNVA, which does not enhance sCT absorption at all (Figure 2). This slow transit was the result of mucoadhesion of nanoparticles (Table I). The mucoadhesion strength of nanoparticles was evaluated by an *in situ* intestinal perfusion technique and it was shown that it depended on the chemical structure of macromonomers on the nanoparticle surface. The mucoadhesion of PNIPAAm nanoparticles was stronger than that of ionic nanoparticles. It seemed that PNVA nanoparticles did not adhere to the GI tract. These findings demonstrated that the mucoadhesion of sCT-loaded nanoparticles is closely related to the enhancement of sCT absorption.

Due to their good bioadhesive properties, polyanhydride copolymers of fumaric and sebacic acids, poly(FA:SA), were used to encapsulate dicumarol into microparticles (80 % of spheres were < 1 μm an the remaining were between 1 and 4 μm) [65,66]. Dicumarol is an anticoagulant drug which has a poor water solubility and an erratic intestinal absorption. The encapsulated dicumarol formulation demonstrated a 57 % increase in the AUC plasma concentration-time curve over a spray-dried unencapsulated drug, and a 112 % increase over an unmicronized stock suspension. Furthermore, encapsulated dicumarol was found to remain in plasma for significantly longer periods (72 h) than with the two other formulations (48 h). The improved pharmacokinetic showed by the dicumarol-loaded microspheres was attributed to their bioadhesive properties which enabled a more intimate contact of these carriers with the intestinal mucosa as well as an increased residence time at the local absorption site of the drug [66,67].

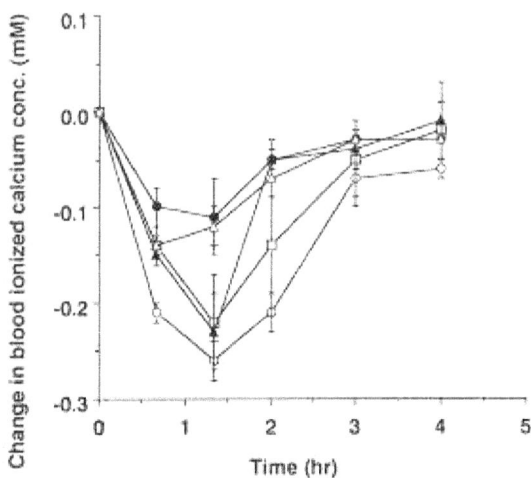

Figure 2. Concentration-time profiles of ionized calcium in blood after oral administration of sCT aqueous solution (●),sCT–PNIPAAm nanoparticles (○),sCTPNVA nanoparticles (△), sCT–PVAm nanoparticles (□) and sCT–PMAA nanoparticles (▲) in rats (0.25 mg sCT with 25 mg nanoparticles in 2.5 ml dosing solution/kg rat). Adapted from reference [54].

Table I. Kinetic parameters in the gastrointestinal tract of polystyrene nanoparticles having surface hydrophilic chains

Formulation of nanoparticles	Gastric empty rate (% of dose/min)	Transit rate through intestinal tract (% of dose/min)
PNIPAAm	0.62	0.39
PNVA	1.42	1.26
PVAm	0.35	0.23
PMAA	0.87	0.44
Control	1.67	1.32

[f] PEG aqueous solution (Mn : 4000)

Also performed by this research group, insulin was encapsulated in mucoadhesive nanoparticles made of a blend of poly(fumaric anhydride) and poly(lactide-*co*-glycolide) 50:50. For the *in vivo* study, fasted rats were first injected with an initial glucose load and then orally administered with different formulations. The blood glucose levels of rats dosed with zinc-insulin-loaded nanoparticles (97 nm) were successfully controlled at the fasting levels (< 5 mg/dl) for at least 5 h. Conversely, rats fed with insulin solution and saline reached maximum blood glucose levels of 36 mg/dl after 1.5 h and 46 mg/ dl after 3 h, respectively. Clearly, animals fed with the encapsulated insulin were better able to regulate the glucose load than the controls [67].

Mucoadhesive poly(D,L-lactide-*co*-gylcolide) nanospheres coated with chitosan were developed in order to improve oral absorption and prolong the physiological activity of elcatonin, a peptide derivate of calcitonin [62]. After intragastric administration to fasted rats, chitosan-coated nanospheres reduced significantly the blood calcium level compared with elcatonin solution and uncoated nanospheres. Moreover, the reduced calcium level was sustained for a period of 48 h. Even under nonfasting conditions, the mucoadhesion of chitosan-coated nanospheres was unaltered and the reduction in blood calcium level was maintained satisfactory.

Arangoa et al. [16] established a correlation of the pharmacokinetic parameters of the carbazole orally administered in gliadin nanoparticles with the *in vivo* bioadhesive properties of these carriers. Two types of bioadhesive carriers were assessed in the study, i.e. non-hardened gliadin nanoparticles (NH-NP) and crosslinked gliadin nanoparticles (CL-NP). The oral absorption of carbazole was highly increased by both nanoparticles leading to bioavailability values of 40 % for NH-NP and 49 % for CL-NP. Moreover, the pharmacokinetic parameters obtained from CL-NP (a lower C_{max}, a higher T_{max} and a smaller k_{el}) suggested that this formulation might provide a sustained release of carbazole. Finally, it was relevant that a good correlation was found between the carbazole plasma levels, during the period of time in which the absorption process prevails, and the amount of adhered nanoparticles (NH-NP as well as CL-NP) to the stomach mucosa (Figure 3). Clearly, the enhancement in the drug absorption was determined by the global balance of two phenomena: the modification in the release pattern of drug and the bioadhesion of nanoparticles, which in turn are influenced by the crosslinking degree of polymer.

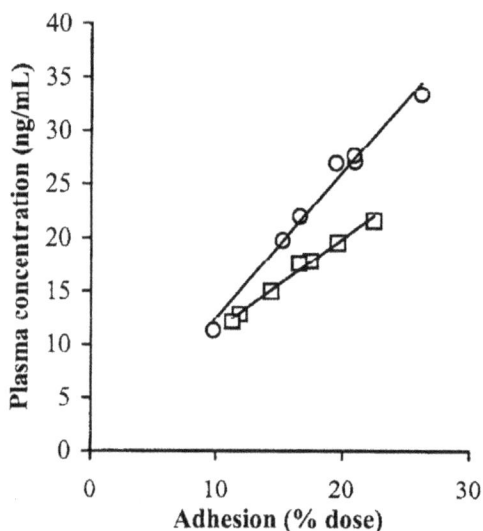

Figure 3. Correlation between the amount of carbazole-loaded
nanoparticles that adhered to the stomach mucosa after oral
administration and their corresponding carbazole plasma
concentrations. Non-hardened gliadin nanoparticles (○) and
crosslinked gliadin nanoparticles (□). Adapted from reference [16] .

Limitations of mucoadhesive nanoparticles for increasing the oral absorption
The above mentioned studies showed that conferring mucoadhesive properties
to nanoparticles result in their prolonged transit time in the GI tract which, in
turn, can lead to enhance the oral absorption of the encapsulated drug.
However, mucoadhesive nanoparticles have certain limitations. First, they
adhere to their substrate by nonspecific interactions which implicates that they

may adhere to surfaces they are not intended for. They cannot distinguish
between adherent or shed-off mucus, or the surfaces of other gut contents (e.g.
food). Premature interaction with other substrates may prevent the nanoparticles
from binding to the mucosal tissue surfaces for which they were targeted to.
Besides to their nonspecificity, it should be pointed out that since the
mucoadhesive systems are bound to the intestinal mucus layer through
interactions with mucin, the transit time of these systems is determined by the
physiological turnover time of the mucus layer. Considering that the mucin
turnover time in rats is between 50 and 270 min, mucoadhesive nanoparticles
are not expected to adhere for more than 4-5 h [68]. In this case, drug release
from nanoparticles should be completed during this period of time. This
constitutes thus a limiting factor for functionality of these mucoadhesive
colloidal carriers in the GI tract. Finally, the coadministration of other drugs
and the characteristics of mucin in disease states should be also considered
[23,69] because both factors could also alter the effectiveness of the
mucoadhesive particulate systems.

Specific bioadhesive drug delivery systems at intestinal level
An alternative for bioadhesive nanoparticles is their adhesion directly to the
surface of the cells of the mucosa. In this case, it is necessary to involve specific
interactions between a receptor present at the cell surface and the nanoparticles.
The binding of bioactive molecules (e.g. lectins or other proteins) to the surface
of nanoparticulate carriers has been proposed to specifically recognize receptors
of cells located within the GI tract.

Lectins are natural proteins or glycoproteins that bind reversibly and specifically
to carbohydrate moieties of complex glycoconjugates. The exact physiological

role of lectins is unknown but they are involved in many cell recognition and adhesion processes. In the pharmaceutical field they have been currently described as "second generation mucoadhesives". In contrast to the mucoadhesive polymers, lectins can specifically recognize receptor-like structures of the cell membrane and therefore would bind directly to the epithelial cells themselves rather than to the mucus gel layer. So, associated to colloidal carriers, lectins may confer bioadhesive properties to particles in order to delay their transit time. Moreover, once the receptor–mediated bioadhesion is achieved, lectins may also trigger the active transport of large molecules or colloidal drug carrier systems by vesicular transport processes (endocytosis or transcytosis) [70,71]. For instance, Arbos and co-workers [72] observed that the covalent binding of *Sambucus nigra* lectin to the surface of nanoparticles increased the residence time of carriers to the gut mucosa of rat following oral administration.

Other *in vitro* and *ex vivo* studies have reported the potential use of lectins conjugated to the surface of nanoparticles as drug targeting systems for the GI tract [73-75]. However, this favorable effect has been proved less obvious *in vivo*. It was observed that, after oral administration to rats, the overall transit of lectin-particles conjugates was markedly delayed, but it was entirely due to retention of particles in the stomach. In addition, particle adhesion to intestinal cells did not appear to be lectin specific. The authors attributed these unfavorable results to the limited capacity of the particles to diffuse through the mucus layer and to premature adsorption of soluble mucus glycoproteins to the conjugates [76]. Regarding the second hypothesis, which seems to be highly probable, several studies have reported a marked interaction between lectins (alone or associated to particles) and mucin [73,74,77-79]. This implies that, *in vivo*, lectin-particle conjugates could simply be bound to the glycoproteins of the GI mucus, transported through the GI tract bound to the mucus and then eliminated in the faeces. As a result, the conjugate could never reach the enterocyte surface. In other words, lectin-conjugates are expected to suffer at least partially from premature inactivation by shed off mucus like bioadhesives of the first generation. In conclusion, the use of lectin conjugates for targeting the GI tract in order to reduce the transit time of pharmaceutical formulations has had limited success. Furthermore, the adverse effects, such as cytotoxicity, inflammation and GI irritation [80,81] as well as immunological effects [82,83] induced by the lectins could also restrict their use for oral drug delivery systems.

Other proteins have been also associated to nanoparticles for inducing a specific biadhesion to the GI tract. Using a rat model, it was determined that the bovine serum albumin coating onto nanoparticles influenced the transit and bioadhesive pattern of these colloids in the GI tract [63,72]. The stomach emptying and intestine rates diminished at least twice in comparison with naked nanoparticles. Indeed, the intensity of the bioadhesive phenomenon was significantly higher than for control [63].

Nanoparticles conjugates with lectins and other bioactive molecules, such as adhesins and invasins, have also been investigated for improving the uptake of nanoparticles in the GI tract. This topic is discussed in Section 4.

3.5.3. Influence of vehicle on the oral absorption of drugs from nanoparticles

Several studies support the importance of the liquid vehicle used to disperse and administer nanoparticles. Using streptozotocin-induced diabetic rats, Damgé et

142

al. [51] observed that the biological response of insulin-loaded nanoparticles depended on the vehicle used for their oral administration. When dispersed in an oily medium (Miglyol 812) containing surfactant agents (poloxamer 188 and deoxycholic acid), nanospheres provoked a 50 % decrease of fasted glycemia from the second hour up to 10-13 days. Conversely, the hypoglycemic effect was shorter (2 h) or absent when nanospheres were dispersed in water with or without surfactants (Figure 4).

Further, based on the fact that microemulsions incorporating medium-chain glycerides can enhance peptide absorption [84,85], Watnasirichaikul et al. [31] evaluated the potential of PBCA nanocapsules dispersed in a microemulsion to promote the absorption of insulin following oral administration to diabetic rats. The microemulsion used as vehicle contained a mixture of medium chain mono-, di-, and tri-glycerides as oil component and polysorbate 80 and sorbitan monooleate as surfactants. Intragastric administration of insulin-loaded nanocapsules dispersed in the microemulsion resulted in greater reduction in blood glucose levels of diabetic rats than an aqueous insulin solution or insulin formulated only in the microemulsion. The authors postulated that the release of insulin in the intestine in presence of the microemulsion excipients could facilitate the intestinal absorption of some of the released insulin before its enzymatic digestion.

In addition, it has been suggested that the vehicle might induce variations in the hydrophilicity/hydrophobicity of the nanoparticle surface and then alter the uptake of these carriers in the GI tract. This topic is discussed in the next Section.

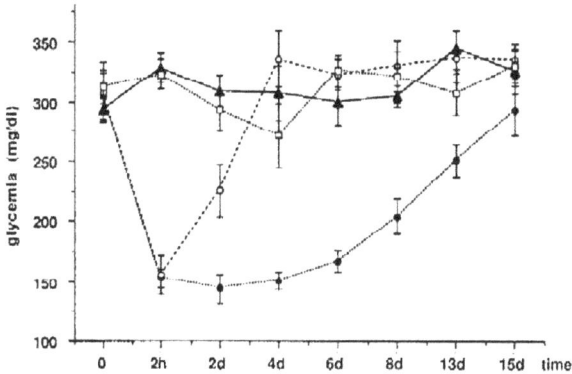

Figure 4. Effect of a single intragastric administration of insulin-loaded nanospheres (100 U/kg) dispersed in water (□), in water containing surfactant agents (1 % poloxamer 188 and 0.01 deoxycholic acid) (○), and Miglyol 812 containing the above mentioned surfactants (●) on glycemia of streptozotocin-induced diabetic rats. Control animals received a peroral administration of 100 U/kg of free insulin in Miglyol 812 containing surfactans (▲); n = 8, mean ± S.E.M. Adapted from reference [51].

4. *In vivo* studies using nanoparticles for oral delivery of vaccines

During the last two decades, intense studies were carried out to assess if transmucosal passage of nanoparticules across the mammalian GI tract is effective and if following their internalisation into the intestinal cells, nanoparticles might be translocated into circulation to eventually deliver their content in the blood, lymph or even target organs [30,86-95]. Since only a very small percentage of administered nanoparticles is apparently taken into the tissues, it was postulated that delivery of drugs by nanoparticles in a target organ would be restricted for the delivery of potent drugs which require low doses for inducing a therapeutic effect [96-98]. Anyways, as proposed by several authors, the intestinal absorption of nanoparticles can be relevant in other medical areas, for example, in the design of delivery systems for inducing oral immunization and gene transfer [96,99-101]. In fact, the oral delivery of macromolecules such as antigens and genes is frequently compromised by their poor uptake which is mainly due to their size and hydrophilicity; it is well known that only a limited amount of intact molecules reaches the circulation because of lumenal, brush border and intracellular degradation. In this context, the encapsulation in nanoparticulate systems may protect these macromolecules from enzymatic degradation, increase their uptake in intact form and potentially target the molecules to the desired sites in the body. Indeed, enhanced responses to orally delivered encapsulated antigens have been reported on a number of occasions [99,102]. Gene delivery has also been reported [101].

4.1 Uptake of polymeric particles across the digestive tract

Several *in vivo* studies have reported the uptake of polystyrene and biodegradable particles from the GI tract. Three possible routes for GI uptake of small particles exist: i) intracellular uptake by enterocytes, and ii) intracellular as well as iii) paracellular transfer or uptake via the M cells of Peyer's patches. These mechanisms seem to take place simultaneously and to occur in different degrees at different sites of the gut. In fact, the dominant opinion appears to suggest that particulate uptake in mammals is principally via the M cells of Peyer's patches. Even though, uptake by enterocytes in the villous part of the

GI tract and particulate transport by a paracellular pathway has been also evidenced by microscopy, these mechanisms probably play an minor role in particle uptake [96,98]. The extent of particle uptake considerably depends on the physicochemical characteristics of the particles such as the size, hydrophobicity, charge, and polymeric composition of the particles.

4.1.1. Factors affecting the extent of uptake of nanoparticles

Size

Particle size is a critical determinant of the fate of orally delivered nanoparticles. The uptake of particles is clearly size-dependent. It is generally accepted that nanoparticles are more efficiently absorbed than microparticles [89,103,104]. Larger particles may be retained for longer periods in the Peyer's patches while smaller particles are progressively transported to other major organs [90].

Jani et al. [89] determined that, after oral administration to rats, polystyrene nanoparticles in the size range of 50 nm to 3 μm showed important levels of interaction with the GI mucosa. Adhesion as well as uptake of nanoparticles corresponded to 30 % of the initial dose of smallest nanoparticles (50 and 100 nm). In particular, about 7 % of the 50 nm particles and 4 % of the 100 nm particles accumulated in the liver, spleen and bone marrow. Histological studies confirmed the extent of nanoparticles distribution and revealed that uptake of nanoparticles occurred through both the gut-associated lymphoid tissue (GALT) and, to a lesser extent, normal intestine tissue [88,90,105]. In addition, the largest particles (3 μm) did not apparently migrate to the liver, spleen and blood [89], but histological observation revealed that these particles were adsorbed and immobilized within the submucosal layer of the thicker mucosa and the Peyer's patches [88,90].

Jenkins et al. [106] also investigated the absorption of particles with different sizes (0.15 to 10.0 µm) from the rat intestine. Specifically, they observed that the levels of absorption, retention and extravasation of nanoparticles was dependent on the particle size. The 0.5 µm nanoparticles were found to be absorbed in significantly greater number by the Peyer's patches and the mesenteric lymph than other sizes; 3.0 µm particles were retained in the mesenteric lymph nodes in greater number than all other particles; and, 10.0 µm particles were retained in the mesenteric lymph nodes in only low numbers.

Using poly(lactic-*co*-glycolic acid) particles (100 nm, 500 nm, 1µm, and 10 µm), Desai et al. [104] investigated the effect of particle size on GI tissue uptake. The efficiency of uptake of 100 nm size particles by the intestinal tissue was 15-250 fold higher compared to larger size particles. Moreover, histological examination of the Peyer's patch and non-patch tissue showed that 100 nm nanoparticles were distributed into the submucosal layers as compared to larger particles which were mostly aligned at the epithelial linings [104]. It seems that particles in the range 3-10 µm are sequestered within the Peyer's patches and do not migrate into the mesenteric lymph nodes [107,108].

Polymer composition
The polymeric composition of particles, in particular its hydrophobicity, is another factor that governs the extent of particle uptake. Eldridge et al. [107] determined that, following oral administration to mice, hydrophobic polystyrene particles were preferentially taken up, poly(lactic acid) and poly(lactide-*co*-

glycolide) particles taken up to a lesser extent, and hydrophilic cellulose matrices were not taken up at all. A study in rabbits has confirmed that polystyrene nanoparticles (500-600 nm) are preferentially taken up over poly(lactide-co-glycolide) nanoparticles [109]. Other studies showed that the adsorption of hydrophilic polymers (poloxamer surfactants) onto polystyrene nanoparticles (50-60 nm) reduced their uptake from the large intestine and inhibited their uptake in the small intestine [91,110,111]. This demonstrates that absorption process is dictated by surface features of nanoparticles. Particle charge is also an important factor which determines the extent of uptake from the gut. A study carried out in rats showed that negatively charged nanoparticles (100 and 1000 nm) were taken up to a lesser degree than the non-ionized particles [88].

Vehicle for administration

The extent of uptake of nanoparticles can be altered by changing the vehicle in which the particles are dispersed. While the oral administration of an aqueous suspension of nanoparticles (133 nm) in mice showed a low percentage of absorption of particles (0.5 %), association of these nanoparticles with concentrated milk slightly increased the amount of absorbed nanoparticles (2.4 %). It was supposed that the lipids contained in the milk could have stimulated the lymphatic absorption of nanoparticles [94]. In another study, when delivered with lecithin, uptake of polystyrene nanoparticles (500 nm) was significantly greater than in the saline controls, whereas with oleic acid, uptake of particles was significantly lower. The different effects of these lipids on the uptake of nanoparticles could be due to the specific interaction of lipids with membranes [97]. The volume and the tonicity of the administration vehicle have also been reported to affect the extent of uptake of polystyrene nanoparticles (817 nm) following oral administration to rats [92]. Finally, it was determined in mice that the intestinal uptake of nanoparticles is also dose dependent [108,112].

Other factors

Physiological factors, which include animal species, age and food ingestion, have also an influence on the uptake mechanism of polymeric nanoparticles. The extent of uptake of nanoparticles in rabbits seems to be at least 1 order of magnitude greater than in mice, probably because of the much greater abundance of M cells in the rabbit Peyer's patches [96,113]. The age as well as a pathological state of the animals also seems to affect particle uptake [87,93,96,112,113]. The presence of food is another enhancing factor for particle uptake, possibly because it increases the intestinal transit time [108,114].

4.1.2. Targeting agents to promote the nanoparticle uptake

Nanoparticle uptake can be not only improved, but also modulated, by coupling specific tissue- or cell- ligands onto the nanoparticle surface. The most common bioactive molecules used for this end include antibodies [115-118], lectins [75,83,119-121] invasins [119,122-124] and Vitamin B12 [119,125,126]. Such bioactive molecules, *per se*, have the ability to adhere to the surface of intestinal cells and, in most cases, they can also stimulate a vesicular transport process by these cells. It is thus expected that ligand-nanoparticule conjugates can follow the same behavior that the ligand itself. Several *in vivo* studies have shown the potential use of these ligand-coupled nanoparticles as oral delivery systems.

Hussain et al. [121] evidenced that up to 23% of tomato lectin-conjugated nanoparticles (500 nm) administered orally to rats for 5 days were translocated into the systemic circulation. This represented a 50-fold increase when compared to the control (hapten-blocked particles) which exhibit less than 0.5 % of systemic absorption. Interestingly, nanoparticles were clearly taken up mainly by the enterocytes, not by the lymphoid tissue (Peyer's patches). Using an everted gut sac model, Carreno-Gomez et al. [127] confirmed that tomato lectin promotes uptake of nanospheres across rat intestine.

Another effort to improve the oral uptake of nanoparticles was focused on utilizing bacterial mechanisms of ephitelial cell entry. Hussain and Florence [124] coupled to the surface of fluorescent latex nanoparticles a truncated form of an outer membrane protein from *Yersinia pseudotuberculosis*. This protein, also termed invasin, is a virulence factor which allows the entry of the pathogen to the intracellular epithelial compartment in order to protect it from the host's immune system. The smaller invasin-C192 moiety, which is by itself capable to promote cellular internalisation, was conjugated to 500 nm nanoparticles. After a single oral dose of a suspension of invasin coupled nanoparticles to rats, it was observed that up to 13 % of the invasin conjugate was present in the systemic circulation. This effect was significantly higher than the controls which attained about 2 % in the blood.

When antibodies were used as specific ligands the results were variable. While some authors reported that coating particles with IgA and IgG increased the uptake by Peyer's patch M cells [116,117], other observed that the association of human immunoglobulin A to nanoparticles (500 nm) did not result in significant selective binding of nanospheres to M-cells [115].

4.2. Oral immunization using nanoparticles

Oral administration of vaccines is desired from both the immunological and patient compliance points of view [101]. Unlike systemic vaccination, oral vaccination avoids the pain and discomfort associated with injections. Because of its non-invasive character, it also eliminates the risk of infections caused by the use of needles and syringes. Moreover, oral vaccination does not require trained personnel for administration. In general, this will lead to better patient compliance and lower cost. Oral administration of vaccines may make large-population immunization more feasible. From an immunological viewpoint, oral delivery of vaccines might also induce both systematic and mucosal immune response. This might prove particularly advantageous because almost all the pathogens causing common infectious diseases enter or infect the body via mucosal surfaces. Thus, proper induction of mucosal immune responses may be useful to prevent infection or onset of disease.

The majority of the GALT is organized into aggregates of lymphoid follicles called Peyer's patches. The major physiological role of the Peyer's patches is the induction of a secretory immune response to ingested antigens. In humans, the largest Peyer's patches are found in the terminal ileum and are covered with a specialized epithelium that is adapted to allow antigen sampling from the lumen. On contact, antigens are then delivered into the underlying dome structures of the patches through specialized cells called M cells. There are two important aspects of the uptake and transport of antigens by M cells: i) antigens will probably escape degradation, and ii) the antigen will be released into an environment rich in immunocompetent cells. Thus uptake by M cells can enable the delivery of intact antigens into the immunoinductive enviroment of the

Peyer's patches. Therefore, knowing that the M cells represents the favored route for nanoparticle uptake, several authors have investigated the use of these particulate systems containing entrapped or adsorbed antigens as vaccine adjuvant alternative.

Among other strategies for oral vaccination, the use of nanoparticles is of interest because these carriers offer potential advantages such as protection of the antigen from degradation in the gut, diminution in the number of inoculations and enhancement of the immune response after oral immunization. Further, experimental animals immunized by PLG-entrapped antigens produce both humoral and cellular immunity and can in some instances be protected from subsequent infection. The ability of these systems for the delivery of complex antigens, combination of antigens [13,128] and recombinant and genetic vaccines [129,130] makes of them one of the most promising strategies for oral vaccination.

4.2.1.   Immune responses following oral immunization with antigen-loaded nanoparticles

Increased levels of systemic antibody have been reported after oral administration of antigen in particulate systems. It has been established that antigen incorporated into nanoparticles are more effective for oral immunization than soluble antigens. The ability of particulate antigens to induce enhanced immune responses following oral immunization is mainly a consequence of their greater uptake into intestinal Peyer's patches.

O'Hagan and co-workers [131-133] showed that oral immunization of mice with ovalbumin (OVA) entrapped in poly(lactide-*co*-glycolide) particles induced potent serum and salivary antibody responses. They also observed that the degradation rate of polymer had an relevant influence on the immune response. The more rapidly degrading polymer was most effective for the induction of high levels of salivary IgA antibodies, while the slowest degrading polymer was most effective for the induction of serum IgG antibodies [133]. Interestingly, subsequent studies by the same group showed that the secretory IgA response was disseminated throughout the common mucosal immune system to the nose, the gut and the lower genital tract [134]. This confirmed the thesis that, by way of the common mucosal immune system, committed lymphocytes migrate from the gut-associated lymphoid tissue to other mucosa-associated lymphoid tissue. Finally, a systemic cytotoxic T lymphocyte response in mouse splenocytes was detected following multiple oral immunizations with OVA-loaded particles [135].

After oral administration to mice of poly(D,L-lactide-*co*-glycolide) particles (1-10 μm) containing staphylococcal enterotoxin B toxoid, circulating toxin-specific antibodies and a concurrent sIgA antitoxin response in saliva were detected. In contrast, the soluble antigen was relatively ineffective as an immunogen following oral administration [107].

Jung et al. [136] investigated the humoral immune response induced by tetanus toxoid-loaded nanoparticles in mice. A charge modified biodegradable polymer, poly(vinyl alcohol)-graft-poly(lactide-*co*-glycolide), was used to reach a high level of antigen loading by adsorption. Tetanus toxoid-loaded nanoparticles given perorally induced serum IgG and IgA immune responses in mice. This effect was significantly increased by the coadministration of cholera toxin adjuvant. Even, the IgA titers were significantly increased compared to the control (i.p. administration). The particle size affected the induction of antibody titers in a significant manner. For oral administration it is likely that smaller nanoparticles induce higher IgA and IgG titers. Furthermore, different doses are needed for the induction of IgG and total serum antibodies titers. An oral dose of 9.4 µg TT associated to nanoparticles is sufficient to induce an IgA response, while 28.9 µg are needed to induce significant increased serum IgG titers.

The adjuvant effect of nanoparticles for the oral route has been compared to the most potent oral adjuvant available, cholera toxin. Depending on the immunization protocol employed, it was shown that cholera toxin B subunit (CTB) entrapped in nanoparticles (420 nm) induced comparable serum and intestinal antibody responses to CTB mixed with cholera toxin [137].

Particle size has a significant effect on the immunogenicity of antigen-loaded nanoparticles. The induction of IgG and IgA antibody responses after oral application is strongly influenced by the particle size distribution. While particles larger than 1 µm did not induce antibody titers at all (similar to pure TT in solution), significant titers were observed after application of 500 nm nanoparticles. The highest antibody titers were found in case of 100 nm [136]. O'Hagan et al. [138] incorporated by adsorption a model antigen, OVA, onto poly(butyl-2-cyanoacrylate) nanoparticles having two different sizes. Oral immunization in rats with OVA-nanoparticles resulted in enhanced antibody responses in comparison to oral immunization with soluble OVA. Moreover, smaller nanoparticles (100 nm) appeared to be more effective than larger particles (3 µm) for the induction of salivary IgA responses. The enhanced efficacy of the smaller particles was probably a consequence of their greater uptake into the Peyer's patches.

In the study carried out by Conway et al. [139], cholera toxin B subunit was adsorbed to the surface of 200 or 1000 nm polystyrene nanospheres and administered orally to mice. Both nanospheres induced systemic immunity in the form of circulating anti-cholera toxin B subunit IgG. Significantly, latex particles of 200 nm induced strongest gut-specific IgA responses, which suggested that submicron particulates access IgA inductive compartments in gut-associated lymphoid tissue to a greater extent than one micron diameter carriers.

Gutierro and co-workers [140] investigated the influence of dose on the serum Ig G antibody response of an antigen entrapped into poly(lactide-*co*-glycolide) nanoparticles following orally administration. By increasing the amount of the encapsulated antigen per dose (from 50 to 200 μg), the immune response also increased up to a level (> 200 μg) at which the serum IgG response did not change. It was also observed that an encapsulated antigen can display more efficiently the Ig G specific response. Antigen-loaded nanoparticles administered by oral route are capable to elicit a combined serum Ig G2a/Ig G1 responses, with a predominance of the Ig G1 antibody. In contrast, soluble antigens usually elicit high levels of Ig G1 antibody isotype, but very low levels of Ig G2a. This result is particularly of interest because Ig G2 is able to act as an opsonin, activates the complement and binds to macrophages for enhancing the phagocytic response.

Chapitre V

Increased systemic antibody levels have been reported after oral administration of antigen in poly(lactide-*co*-glycolide) microparticles. The adsorption of antigen onto biodegradable particles has been shown to enhance secretory immune responses in comparison with soluble antigen in gastrically immunized rats. This indicates that poly(lactide-*co*-glycolide) particles exert an adjuvant effect not entirely dependent on antigen entrapment.

4.2.2. Protective immunity following oral immunization with antigen-loaded nanoparticles

While the aforementioned reports give evidences that oral administration of antigens with nanoparticles could be a highly effective means of inducing immune responses, to date only a handful of workers have reported the protection induced by antigen-loaded nanoparticles against a number of pathogens.

Oral immunization with fimbriae from *Bordetella pertussis* entrapped in nanoparticles (2000 nm) protected mice from intranasal challenge with the pathogen [141]. In addition, the encapsulated fimbriae orally administered elicited not only disseminated mucosal immune responses but also systemic immune responses, which are comparable to those elicited by i.p. injection of encapsulated fimbriae. Oral immunization with the encapsulated antigen gave rise to specific IgA and IgG responses in saliva, stools and vaginal washings. The demonstration that a single oral dose of encapsulated *B. pertussis* fimbria confers protection at remote mucosal surfaces is testimony that, for certain antigens, oral vaccination has enormous potential.

156

In another study, a hot saline extract (HS) from *Brucella ovis* was encapsulated in poly-ε-caprolactone nanoparticles (1400 nm). After oral administration to mice, HS-NP protected the animals against *B. ovis* infection. Such protection was similar to that provided by the reference living attenuated *B. melitensis* Rev. 1 vaccine. By contrast, oral vaccination with HS nanoparticles did not confer protection against *B. abortus* infection to mice [142].

The immunogenicity and protective efficacy of orally delivered pertussis antigens entrapped in particulate formulations were evaluated in a murine respiratory challenge model for infection with *Bordetella pertussis*. For this end, two protective antigens from *B. pertussis*, pertussis toxoid (PTd) and filamentous haemagglutinin (FHA), were encapsulated in PLG microparticles (2.7 μm) or nanoparticles (350 nm); blends of the two PLG particulates were administered to mice in order to induce the immune response. Substantial IgG serum titers were generated following oral immunization with PTd and FHA encapsulated in microparticles or nanoparticles. Furthermore, oral administration of encapsulated antigens induced secretory IgA in lungs of mice following infection with *B. pertussis*. Encapsulated antigens efficiently protected mice against the pathogen: there was a reduction in the levels of bacteria in lungs at 10-14 days after the challenge and no viable *B. pertussis* were detected in lungs after day 14. In addition, the level of protection observed following oral delivery of pertussis antigens in nanoparticles approached that observed with systemic delivery, albeit using 20 to 100 fold higher doses and three immunizations [143]. Finally, these findings showed that, although further progress is necessary to reduce the dose of antigen required, oral administration of encapsulated vaccines is possible.

4.2.3. DNA encapsulation into nanoparticles for oral vaccination

Using DNA vaccines (i.e. DNA plasmids that code for antigenic proteins) the antigen is synthesized in vivo directly from the protein-coding sequences. An advantage of this approach compared with the conventional attenuated-vaccine approach is that the vector is unlikely to become pathogenic. In addition, antigenic competition with the vector should not arise. Recent studies have shown that polymeric nanoparticulate carriers can be used for the oral delivery of DNA. Entrapping DNA plasmids in nanoparticles combines the concept of mucosal vaccination with that of DNA vaccination. Studies have shown that plasmid DNA can be encapsulated in nanoparticles with significant retention of biological function, and an oral dose of encapsulated DNA can elicit systemic and mucosal antibody responses to the encoded protein.

Jones et al. [129] encapsulated a plasmid-expressing insect luciferase protein into PLGA nanoparticles (2000 nm) and administered it to mice by oral gavage. They observed good serum IgG, IgA and IgM antibody responses, and most importantly, significant levels of mucosal IgA in saliva and stool samples. In contrast, unencapsulated pDNA gave much weaker responses. Cellular immune responses, however, were not characterized.

Using poly(lactide-*co*-glycolide) nanoparticles containing rotavirus VP6 DNA vaccine, Chen et al. [144] reported that one dose of vaccine given to BALB/c mice elicited both rotavirus-specific serum antibodies and intestinal IgA. Moreover, after challenge with homologous rotaviruses, virus shedding was significantly reduced compared to control mice, which were immunized with nanoparticles containing VP6-free plasmid. Similar results were observed when

VP6 gene was replaced with VP4 and /or VP7 [145]. These findings demonstrated the protection against an infectious agent elicited after oral administration of DNA vaccines.

Chitosan nanoparticles constitute a further type of carriers that has demonstrated efficacy for the oral administration of vaccines. As showed by Roy et al. [130], oral gene delivery with high-molecular-weight (390 kDa) chitosan-DNA nanoparticles resulted in an immunological protection in a mouse model of peanut allergy. Mice receiving nanoparticles containing a dominant peanut allergen gene produced secretory IgA and serum IgG_{2a}. Compared with non-immunized mice or those treated only with naked DNA, mice immunized with chitosan nanoparticles showed a substantial reduction in allergen-induced anaphylaxis associated with reduced levels of IgE, plasma histamine and vascular leakage. To assess the expression and distribution of transduced gene, prior oral administration of chitosan particles complexed with plasmid encoding for β-galactosidase resulted in only the epithelial cells of both the stomach and particularly the small intestine to be stained with x-gal, a substrate for the enzyme. Encouragingly, 10% of the entire epithelium was stained although no mention of PP was made. No underlying immune cells were stained suggesting that the 200 nm particles were unable to traffic across the cell interior. By contrast, preliminary results from Koping-Hoggard et al. [146] demonstrate only a small but significant gene expression upon oral administration in mice with chitosan–DNA complexes of lower positive zeta potential compared to DNA condensed with the highly charged non-biodegradable polyethyleimine cationic polymer.

Other biodegradable materials for encapsulating plasmid DNA have also shown promise in oral delivery of DNA. Expression levels in rat PP, intestine and liver fed with poly(fumaric-*co*-sebacic) incorporating plasmid DNA encoding for β-galactosidase increased twofold compared to oral administration of naked plasmid [67].

5. Conclusions and perspectives

Critical examination of *in vivo* studies presented in this review show that association of active molecules with nanoparticles can result in favorable results when orally administered. Nanoparticles have shown to be efficient not only for improving the pharmacological local activity of drugs in the GI tract, but also for enhancing the oral absorption and systemic response of active compounds. Moreover, the oral administration of nanoparticles may promote favorable therapeutic aspects such as reduction of adverse effects of compounds in the GI tract, diminution of interindividual variability of the pharmacological response of drugs. Likewise, several studies have evidenced that polymeric nanoparticles can be efficient delivery systems for oral vaccination.

Although these observations suggest a high potential for nanoparticles as oral drug delivery system, some factors have limited the development oral formulations based on nanoparticles. One primary concerns the possible instability of some labile compounds (e.g. peptides, proteins and genes) incorporated into nanoparticles. During nanoparticle preparation, inactivation of protein could occur due to exposure to organic solvents and high shear forces. Second, the acidic environment generated during the degradation of PLGA matrix due to the formation of acidic monomers and oligomers could produce a degradation of protein. Moreover, pharmacological, pharmaceutical and technological aspects should be considered. Requirements for introduction into a market of an oral formulation based on nanoparticles should include: low dose/frequency, high safety profile, effective biological effect, physical and chemical stability, and possibility for produce at industrial scale. The future of nanoparticles as oral delivery systems will depend on the advances and efforts achieved in these different fields during the coming years.

References

[1] J. Kreuter, U. Muller, K. Munz, Quantitative and microautoradiographic study on mouse intestinal distribution of polycyanoacrylate nanoparticles, Int. J. Pharm. 55 (1989) 39-45.

[2] A. Dembri, M. J. Montisci, J. C. Gantier, H. Chacun, G. Ponchel, Targeting of 3'-azido 3'-deoxythymidine (AZT)-loaded poly(isohexylcyanoacrylate) nanospheres to the gastrointestinal mucosa and associated lymphoid tissues, Pharm. Res. 18 (2001) 467-473.

[3] C. Damge, M. Aprahamian, G. Balboni, A. Hoeltzel, V. Andrieu, J. P. Devissaguet, Polyalkylcyanoacrylate nanocapsules increase the intestinal absorption of a lipophilic drug, Int. J. Pharm. 36 (1987) 121-125.

[4] B. Hubert, J. Atkinson, M. Guerret, M. Hoffman, J. P. Devissaguet, P. Maincent, The preparation and acute antihypertensive effects of a nanocapsular form of darodipine, a dihydropyridine calcium entry blocker, Pharm. Res. 8 (1991) 734-738.

[5] J. P. Lowe, C. S. Temple, Calcitonin and insulin in isobutylcyanoacrylate nanocapsules: protection against proteases and effect on intestinal absorption in rats, J. Pharm. Pharmacol. 46 (1994) 547-552.

[6] T. Niwa, H. Takeuchi, T. Hino, M. Nohara, Y. Kawashima, Biodegradable submicron carriers for peptide drugs: Preparation of D,L-lactide/glycolide copolymer (PLGA) nanospheres with nafarelin acetate by a novel emulsion-phase separation method in an oil system, Int. J. Pharm. 121 (1995) 45-54.

[7]   S. Sakuma, N. Suzuki, R. Sudo, K. Hiwatari, A. Kishida, M. Akashi, Optimized chemical structure of nanoparticles as carriers for oral delivery of salmon calcitonin, Int. J. Pharm. 239 (2002) 185-195.

[8]   S. Galindo-Rodríguez, E. Allémann, E. Doelker, H. Fessi, Versatility of three techniques for preparing nanoparticles of different sizes and drug loadings, J. Drug Deliv. Sci. Technol. Submitted.

[9]   A. M. Hillery, I. Toth, A. J. Shaw, A. T. Florence, Co-polymerised peptide particles (CPP) I: synthesis, characterisation and in vitro studies on a novel oral nanoparticulate delivery system, J. Control. Release 41 (1996) 271-281.

[10] N. Hussain, A. T. Florence, Invasin-induced oral uptake of nanospheres: utilising bacterial mechanisms of epithelial cell entry, J. Control. Release 41 (1996) S3-S4.

[11] J. M. Anderson, M. S. Shive, Biodegradation and biocompatibility of PLA and PLGA microspheres, Adv. Drug Deliv. Rev. 28 (1997) 5-24.

[12] S. Y. Lin, K. S. Chen, H. H. Teng, M. J. Li, In vitro degradation and dissolution behaviours of microspheres prepared by three low molecular weight polyesters, J. Microencapsul. 17 (2000) 577-586.

[13] A. Prokop, E. Kozlov, G. W. Newman, M. J. Newman, Water-based nanoparticulate polymeric system for protein delivery: permeability control and vaccine application, Biotechnol. Bioeng. 78 (2002) 459-466.

[14] D. P. Callender, N. Jayaprakash, A. Bell, V. Petraitis, R. Petratienes, M. Candelario, R. Schaufele, J. M. Dunn, S. Sei, T. J. Walsh, F. M. Balis, Pharmacokinetics of oral zidovudine entrapped in biodegradable nanospheres in rabbits, Antimicrob. Agents Chemother. 43 (1999) 972-974.

[15] J. M. Dunn, A. S. Hollister, Oral biovailability of heparin using a novel delivery system, Curr. Ther. Res. 56 (1995) 738-745.

[16] M. A. Arangoa, M. A. Campanero, M. J. Renedo, G. Ponchel, J. M. Irache, Gliadin nanoparticles as carriers for the oral administration of lipophilic drugs. Relationships between bioadhesion and pharmacokinetics, Pharm. Res. 18 (2001) 1521-1527.

[17] D. Scherer, F. C. Mooren, R. K. H. Kinne, J. Kreuter, In vitro permeability of PBCA nanoparticles through porcine small intestine., J. Drug. Target. 1 (1993) 21-27.

[18] J. C. Leroux, R. Cozens, J. L. Roesel, B. Galli, F. Kubel, E. Doelker, R. Gurny, Pharmacokinetics of a novel HIV-1 protease inhibitor incorporated into biodegradable or enteric nanoparticles following intravenous and oral administration to mice, J. Pharm. Sci. 84 (1995) 1387-1391.

[19] J. C. Leroux, R. M. Cozens, J. L. Roesel, B. Galli, E. Doelker, R. Gurny, pH-sensitive nanoparticles: an effective means to improve the oral delivery of HIV-1 protease inhibitors in dogs, Pharm. Res. 13 (1996) 485-487.

[20] F. De Jaeghere, E. Allémann, F. Kubel, B. Galli, R. Cozens, E. Doelker, R. Gurny, Oral bioavailability of a poorly water soluble HIV-1 protease inhibitor incorporated into pH-sensitive particles: effect of the particle size and nutritional state, J. Control. Release 68 (2000) 291-298.

[21] R. Bodmeier, H. G. Chen, O. Paeratakul, A novel approach to the oral delivery of micro- or nanoparticles, Pharm. Res. 6 (1989) 413-417.

[22] Y. Akiyama, N. Nagahara, T. Kashihara, S. Hirai, H. Toguchi, *In vitro* and *in vivo* evaluation of mucoadhesive microspheres prepared for the gastrointestinal tract using polyglycerol esters of fatty acids and a poly(acrylic acid) derivative, Pharm. Res. 12 (1995) 397-405.

[23] A. Lamprecht, U. Schafer, C. M. Lehr, Size-dependent bioadhesion of micro- and nanoparticulate carriers to the inflamed colonic mucosa, Pharm. Res. 18 (2001) 788-793.

[24] S. McClean, E. Prosser, E. Meehan, D. O'Malley, N. Clarke, Z. Ramtoola, D. Brayden, Binding and uptake of biodegradable poly-D,L-lactide micro- and nanoparticles in intestinal epithelia, Eur. J. Pharm. Sci. 6 (1998) 153-163.

[25] P. Couvreur, Polyalkylcyanoacrylates as colloidal drug carriers, Crit. Rev. Ther. Drug Carrier Syst. 5 (1988) 1-20.

[26] R. N. Rowland, J. F. Woodley, The stability of liposomes in vitro to pH, bile salts and pancreatic lipase, BBA - Lipids Lipid Met. 620 (1980) 400-409.

[27] C. Chia-Ming, N. Weiner, Gastrointestinal uptake of liposomes. I. *In vitro* and *in situ* studies, Int. J. Pharm. 37 (1987) 75-85.

[28] C. Schmidt, R. Bodmeier, Incorporation of polymeric nanoparticles into solid dosage forms, J. Control. Release 57 (1999) 115-125.

Chapitre V

[29] S. Galindo-Rodríguez, E. Allémann, H. Fessi, E. Doelker, Physicochemical parameters associated with nanoparticle formation in the salting-out, emulsification-diffusion, and nanoprecipitation methods, Pharm. Res. 21 (2004) 1428-1439.

[30] L. Araujo, M. Sheppard, R. Lobenberg, J. Kreuter, Uptake of PMMA nanoparticles from the gastrointestinal tract after oral administration to rats: modification of the body distribution after suspension in surfactant solutions and in oil vehicles, Int. J. Pharm. 176 (1999) 209-224.

[31] S. Watnasirichaikul, T. Rades, G. Tucker, N. M. Davies, In vitro release and oral bioactivity of insulin in diabetic rats using nanocapsules dispersed in biocompatible microemulsion, J. Pharm. Pharmacol. 54 (2002) 473-480.

[32] F. De Jaeghere, E. Doelker, R. Gurny, Nanoparticles, in: E.Mathiowitz (Ed.), Encyclopedia of Controlled Drug Delivery, John Wiley, U. S. A., 1st ed, 1999, pp. 641-664.

[33] K. S. Soppimath, T. M. Aminabhavi, A. R. Kulkarni, W. E. Rudzinski, Biodegradable polymeric nanoparticles as drug delivery devices, J. Control. Release 70 (2001) 1-20.

[34] P. Couvreur, G. Barratt, E. Fattal, P. Legrand, C. Vauthier, Nanocapsule technology: a review, Crit. Rev. Ther. Drug Carrier Syst. 19 (2002) 99-134.

[35] A. De Labouret, O. Thioune, H. Fessi, J. P. Devissaguet, F. Puisieux, Application of an original process for obtaining colloidal dispersions of some coating polymers: preparation, characterization, industrial scale-up, Drug Dev. Ind. Pharm. 21 (1995) 229-241.

[36] A. P. Colombo, S. Briancon, J. Lieto, H. Fessi, Project, design, and use of a pilot plant for nanocapsule production, Drug Dev. Ind. Pharm. 27 (2001) 1063-1072.

[37] F. J. Galan Valdivia, J. A. Vallet Mas, M. V. W. Bergamini. Process of continuous preparation of disperse colloidal systems in the form of nanocapsules or nanoparticles. U.S.A. Patent 5,705,196, (1998).

[38] S. A. Galindo-Rodríguez, F. Puel, S. Briancon, E. Allémann, E. Doelker, H. Fessi, Comparative scale-up of three methods for producing ibuprofen-loaded nanoparticles, Eur. J. Pharm. Sci. Submitted.

[39] P. H. Beck, J. Kreuter, W. E. G. Muller, W. Schatton, Improved peroral delivery of avarol with polybutylcyanoacrylate nanoparticles, Eur. J. Pharm. Biopharm. 40 (1994) 134-137.

[40] S. Sakuma, N. Suzuki, H. Kikuchi, K. i. Hiwatari, K. Arikawa, A. Kishida, M. Akashi, Absorption enhancement of orally administered salmon calcitonin by polystyrene nanoparticles having poly(N-isopropylacrylamide) branches on their surfaces, Int. J. Pharm. 158 (1997) 69-78.

[41] P. Couvreur, V. Lenaerts, B. Kante, M. Roland, P. Speiser, Oral and parenteral administration of insulin associated to hydrolysable nanoparticles, Acta Pharm. Technol. 26 (1980) 220-222.

[42] N. Ammoury, M. Dubrasquet, H. Fessi, J. P. Devissaguet, F. Puisieux, S. Benita, Idomethacin-loaded poly(D,L-lactide) nanocapsules: protection from gastrointestinal ulcerations and anti-inflammatory activity evaluation in rats, Clin. Mater. 13 (1993) 121-130.

[43] S. S. Guterres, H. Fessi, G. Barratt, F. Puisieux, J. P. Devissaguet, Poly(D,L-lactide) nanocapsules containing non-steroidal anti- inflammatory drugs: gastrointestinal tolerance following intravenous and oral administration, Pharm. Res. 12 (1995) 1545-1547.

[44] C. Damge, C. Michel, M. Aprahamian, P. Couvreur, J. P. Devissaguet, Nanocapsules as carriers for oral peptide delivery, J. Control. Release 13 (1990) 233-239.

[45] S. Sakuma, Y. Ishida, R. Sudo, N. Suzuki, H. Kikuchi, K. Hiwatari, A. Kishida, M. Akashi, M. Hayashi, Stabilization of salmon calcitonin by polystyrene nanoparticles having surface hydrophilic polymeric chains, against enzymatic degradation, Int. J. Pharm. 159 (1997) 181-189.

[46] M. Tobio, A. Sanchez, A. Vila, I. Soriano, C. Evora, J. L. Vila-Jato, M. J. Alonso, The role of PEG on the stability in digestive fluids and *in vivo* fate of PEG-PLA nanoparticles following oral administration, Colloids Surf. B 18 (2000) 315-323.

[47] J. Nelson, C. Reynolds-Kohler, W. Margaretten, C. Wiley, C. Reese, J. Levy, Human immunodeficiency virus detected in bowel epithelium from patients with gastrointestinal symptoms, Lancet 331 (1988) 259-262.

Chapitre V

[48] N. Ammoury, H. Fessi, J. P. Devissaguet, M. Dubrasquet, S. Benita, Jejunal absorption, pharmacological activity, and pharmacokinetic evaluation of indomethacin-loaded poly(d,l-lactide) and poly(isobutyl-cyanoacrylate) nanocapsules in rats, Pharm. Res. 8 (1991) 101-105.

[49] R. Pandey, A. Zahoor, S. Sharma, G. K. Khuller, Nanoparticle encapsulated antitubercular drugs as a potential oral drug delivery system against murine tuberculosis, Tuberculosis 83 (2003) 373-378.

[50] P. Sai, C. Damge, A. S. Rivereau, A. Hoeltzel, E. Gouin, Prophylactic oral administration of metabolically active insulin entrapped in isobutylcyanoacrylate nanocapsules reduces the incidence of diabetes in nonobese diabetic mice, J. Autoimmun. 9 (1996) 713-721.

[51] C. Damge, H. Vranckx, P. Balschmidt, P. Couvreur, Poly(alkyl cyanoacrylate) nanospheres for oral administration of insulin, J. Pharm. Sci. 86 (1997) 1403-1409.

[52] D. Scherer, J. R. Robinson, J. Kreuter, Influence of enzymes on the stability of polybutylcyanoacrylate nanoparticles, Int. J. Pharm. 101 (1994) 165-168.

[53] S. Sakuma, N. Suzuki, H. Kikuchi, K. Hiwatari, K. Arikawa, A. Kishida, M. Akashi, Oral peptide delivery using nanoparticles composed of novel graft copolymers having hydrophobic backbone and hydrophilic branches, Int. J. Pharm. 149 (1997) 93-106.

[54] S. Sakuma, M. Hayashi, M. Akashi, Design of nanoparticles composed of graft copolymers for oral peptide delivery, Adv. Drug Deliv. Rev. 47 (2001) 21-37.

[55] A. Vila, A. Sanchez, M. Tobio, P. Calvo, M. J. Alonso, Design of biodegradable particles for protein delivery, J. Control. Release 78 (2002) 15-24.

[56] G. Ponchel, J. M. Irache, Specific and non-specific bioadhesive particulate systems for oral delivery to the gastrointestinal tract, Adv. Drug Deliv. Rev. 34 (1998) 191-219.

[57] H. Takeuchi, H. Yamamoto, Y. Kawashima, Mucoadhesive nanoparticulate systems for peptide drug delivery, Adv. Drug Deliv. Rev. 47 (2001) 39-54.

[58] G. Ponchel, M. J. Montisci, A. Dembri, C. Durrer, D. Duchene, Mucoadhesion of colloidal particulate systems in the gastro-intestinal tract, Eur. J. Pharm. Biopharm. 44 (1997) 25-31.

[59] H. Luessen, J. C. Verhoef, A. G. de Boer, H. E. Junginger, B. J. de Leeuw, G. Borchard, C. M. Lehr, Multifunctional polymers for the peroral delivery of peptide drugs, in: E. Mathiowitz, D. E. Chickering, C. M. Lehr (Eds.), Bioadhesive Drug Delivery Systems - Fundamentals, Novel Approaches, and Development, Marcel Dekker, Inc., New York, U.S.A., 1st ed, 1999, pp. 299-339.

[60] C. Durrer, J. M. Irache, F. Puisieux, D. Duchene, G. Ponchel, Mucoadhesion of latexes. II. Adsorption isotherms and desorption studies, Pharm. Res. 11 (1994) 680-683.

[61] C. Pimienta, F. Chouinard, A. Labib, V. Lenaerts, Effect of various poloxamer coatings on *in vitro* adhesion of isohexylcyanoacrylate nanospheres to rat ileal segments under liquid flow, Int. J. Pharm. 80 (1992) 1-8.

[62] Y. Kawashima, H. Yamamoto, H. Takeuchi, Y. Kuno, Mucoadhesive D,L-lactide/glycolide copolymer nanospheres coated with chitosan to improve oral delivery of elcatonin, Pharm. Dev. Technol. 5 (2000) 77-85.

[63] P. Arbos, M. A. Campanero, M. A. Arangoa, M. J. Renedo, J. M. Irache, Influence of the surface characteristics of PVM/MA nanoparticles on their bioadhesive properties, J. Control. Release 89 (2003) 19-30.

[64] S. Sakuma, R. Sudo, N. Suzuki, H. Kikuchi, M. Akashi, M. Hayashi, Mucoadhesion of polystyrene nanoparticles having surface hydrophilic polymeric chains in the gastrointestinal tract, Int. J. Pharm. 177 (1999) 161-172.

[65] G. Carino, C. Santos, C. J. Chen, E. Mathiowitz, A radiographic study of intestinal transit times of various spray-dried polymer microspheres, Proc. 22nd Int. Symp. Control. Release Bioact. Mater., pp. 314-315 (1995).

[66] D. Chickering, J. Jacob, E. Mathiowitz, Poly(fumaric-*co*-sebacic) microspheres as oral drug delivery systems, Biotechnol. Bioeng. 52 (1996) 96-101.

[67] E. Mathiowitz, J. S. Jacob, Y. S. Jong, G. P. Carino, D. E. Chickering, P. Chaturvedl, C. A. Santos, K. Vljyaraghavan, S. Montgomery, M. Bassett, C. Morrel, Biologically erodable microspheres as potential oral drug delivery systems, Nature 386 (1997) 410-414.

[68] C. M. Lehr, F. G. J. Poelma, H. E. Junginger, J. J. Tukker, An estimate of turnover time of intestinal mucus gel layer in the rat *in situ* loop, Int. J. Pharm. 70 (1991) 235-240.

[69] B. J. Campbell, Biochemical and functional aspects of mucus and mucin-type glycoproteins, in: E. Mathiowitz, D. E. Chickering, C. M. Lehr (Eds.), Bioadhesive Drug Delivery Systems - Fundamentals, Novel Approaches, and Development, Marcel Dekker, Inc., New York, U.S.A., 1st ed, 1999, pp. 85-130.

[70] C. M. Lehr, Lectin-mediated drug delivery: the second generation of bioadhesives, J. Control. Release 65 (2000) 19-29.

[71] C. Bies, C. M. Lehr, J. F. Woodley, Lectin-mediated drug targeting: history and applications, Adv. Drug Deliv. Rev. 56 (2004) 425-435.

[72] P. Arbos, M. A. Arangoa, M. A. Campanero, J. M. Irache, Quantification of the bioadhesive properties of protein-coated PVM/MA nanoparticles, Int. J. Pharm. 242 (2002) 129-136.

[73] C. M. Lehr, J. A. Bouwstra, W. Kok, A. B. Noach, A. G. de Boer, H. E. Junginger, Bioadhesion by means of specific binding of tomato lectin, Pharm. Res. 9 (1992) 547-553.

[74] J. M. Irache, C. Durrer, D. Duchene, G. Ponchel, Bioadhesion of lectin-latex conjugates to rat intestinal mucosa, Pharm. Res. 13 (1996) 1716-1719.

[75] G. J. Russell-Jones, H. Veitch, L. Arthur, Lectin-mediated transport of nanoparticles across Caco-2 and OK cells, Int. J. Pharm. 190 (1999) 165-174.

[76] M. J. Montisci, A. Dembri, G. Giovannuci, H. Chacun, D. Duchene, G. Ponchel, Gastrointestinal transit and mucoadhesion of colloidal suspensions of *Lycopersicon esculentum L.* and *Lotus tetragonolobus* lectin-PLA microsphere conjugates in rats, Pharm. Res. 18 (2001) 829-837.

[77] B. Naisbett, J. Woodley, The potential use of tomato lectin for oral drug delivery: 3. Bioadhesion *in vivo*, Int. J. Pharm. 114 (1995) 227-236.

[78] J. M. Irache, C. Durrer, D. Duchene, G. Ponchel, *In vitro* study of lectin-latex conjugates for specific bioadhesion, J. Control. Release 31 (1994) 181-188.

[79] M. Wirth, K. Gerhardt, C. Wurm, F. Gabor, Lectin-mediated drug delivery: influence of mucin on cytoadhesion of plant lectins *in vitro*, J. Control. Release 79 (2002) 183-191.

[80] J. D. Smart, C. Banchonglikitkul, R. V. Gibbs, S. J. Donovan, D. J. Cook, Lectins in drug delivery to the oral cavity, *in vitro* toxicity studies, S. T. P. Pharma Sciences 13 (2003) 37-40.

[81] J. D. Smart, Lectin-mediated drug delivery in the oral cavity, Adv. Drug Deliv. Rev. 56 (2004) 481-489.

[82] B. Naisbett, J. Woodley, The potential use of tomato lectin for oral drug delivery: 4. Immunological consequences, Int. J. Pharm. 120 (1995) 247-254.

[83] F. Gabor, E. Bogner, A. Weissenboeck, M. Wirth, The lectin-cell interaction and its implications to intestinal lectin-mediated drug delivery, Adv. Drug Deliv. Rev. 56 (2004) 459-480.

[84] W. A. Ritschel, Microemulsions for improved peptide absorption from the gastrointestinal tract, Method. Find. Exp. Clin. Pharmacol. 13 (1991) 205-220.

[85] P. P. Constantinides, J. P. Scalart, C. Lancaster, J. Marcello, G. Marks, H. Ellens, P. L. Smith, Formulation and intestinal absorption enhancement evaluation of water-in-oil microemulsions incorporating medium-chain glycerides, Pharm. Res. 11 (1994) 1385-1390.

[86] M. Nefzger, J. Kreuter, R. Voges, E. Liehl, R. Czok, Distribution and elimination of polymethyl methacrylate nanoparticles after peroral administration to rats, J. Pharm. Sci. 73 (1984) 1309-1311.

[87] M. E. LeFevre, A. M. Boccio, D. D. Joel, Intestinal uptake of fluorescent microspheres in young and aged mice, Proc. Soc. Exp. Biol. Med. 190 (1989) 23-27.

[88] P. Jani, G. W. Halbert, J. Langridge, A. T. Florence, The uptake and translocation of latex nanospheres and microspheres after oral administration to rats, J. Pharm. Pharmacol. 41 (1989) 809-812.

[89] P. Jani, G. W. Halbert, J. Langridge, A. T. Florence, Nanoparticle uptake by the rat gastrointestinal mucosa: quantitation and particle size dependency, J. Pharm. Pharmacol. 42 (1990) 821-826 .

[90] P. U. Jani, A. T. Florence, D. E. McCarthy, Further histological evidence of the gastrointestinal absorption of polystyrene nanospheres in the rat, Int. J. Pharm. 84 (1992) 245-252.

[91] A. T. Florence, A. M. Hillery, N. Hussain, P. U. Jani, Factors affecting the oral uptake and translocation of polystyrene nanoparticles: histological and analytical evidence, J. Drug. Target. 3 (1995) 65-70.

[92] J. Eyles, O. Alpar, W. N. Field, D. A. Lewis, M. Keswick, The transfer of polystyrene microspheres from the gastrointestinal tract to the circulation after oral administration in the rat, J. Pharm. Pharmacol. 47 (1995) 561-565.

[93] L. H. McMinn, G. M. Hodges, K. E. Carr, Gastrointestinal uptake and translocation of microparticles in the streptozotocin-diabetic rat, J. Anat. 189 (Pt 3) (1996) 553-559.

[94] A. M. Le Ray, M. Vert, J. C. Gautier, J. P. Benoit, Fate of [14 C] poly(D,L-lactide-co-glycolide) nanoparticles after intravenous and oral administration to mice, Int. J. Pharm. 106 (1994) 201-211.

[95] C. Damge, M. Aprahamian, H. Marchais, J. P. Benoit, M. Pinget, Intestinal absorption of PLAGA microspheres in the rat, J. Anat. 189 (Pt 3) (1996) 491-501.

[96] E. C. Lavelle, S. Sharif, N. W. Thomas, J. Holland, S. S. Davis, The importance of gastrointestinal uptake of particles in the design of oral delivery systems, Adv. Drug Deliv. Rev. 18 (1995) 5-22.

[97] N. W. Thomas, P. G. Jenkins, K. A. Howard, M. W. Smith, E. C. Lavelle, J. Holland, S. S. Davis, Particle uptake and translocation across epithelial membranes, J. Anat. 189 (Pt 3) (1996) 487-490.

[98] A. T. Florence, The oral absorption of micro- and nanoparticulates: neither exceptional nor unusual, Pharm. Res. 14 (1997) 259-266.

[99] D. T. O'Hagan, Microparticles and polymers for the mucosal delivery of vaccines, Adv. Drug Deliv. Rev. 34 (1998) 305-320.

[100] A. T. Florence, N. Hussain, Transcytosis of nanoparticle and dendrimer delivery systems: evolving vistas, Adv. Drug Deliv. Rev. 50 (2001) S69-S89.

[101] Z. Cui, R. J. Mumper, Microparticles and nanoparticles asdelivery systems for DNA vaccines, Crit. Rev. Ther. Drug Carrier Syst. 20 (2003) 103-137.

[102] H. O. Alpar, J. E. Eyles, E. D. Williamson, Oral and nasal immunization with microencapsulated clinically relevant proteins, S. T. P. Pharma Sciences 8 (1998) 31-39.

[103] G. M. Hodges, E. A. Carr, R. A. Hazzard, C. O'Reilly, K. E. Carr, A commentary on morphological and quantitative aspects of microparticle translocation across the gastrointestinal mucosa, J. Drug Target. 3 (1995) 57-60.

[104] M. P. Desai, V. Labhasetwar, G. L. Amidon, R. J. Levy, Gastrointestinal uptake of biodegradable microparticles: effect of particle size, Pharm. Res. 13 (1996) 1838-1845.

[105] A. M. Hillery, P. U. Jani, A. T. Florence, Comparative, quantitative study of lymphoid and non-lymphoid uptake of 60 nm polystyrene particles, J. Drug. Target. 2 (1994) 151-156.

[106] P. G. Jenkins, K. A. Howard, N. W. Blackball, N. W. Thomas, S. S. Davis, D. T. O'Hagan, Microparticulate absorption from the rat intestine, J. Control. Release 29 (1994) 339-350.

[107] J. H. Eldridge, C. J. Hammond, J. A. Meulbroek, J. K. Staas, R. M. Gilley, T. R. Tice, Controlled vaccine release in the gut-associated lymphoid tissues. I. Orally administered biodegradable microspheres target the peyer's patches, J. Control. Release 11 (1990) 205-214.

[108] J. P. Ebel, A method for quantifying particle absorption from the small intestine of the mouse, Pharm. Res. 7 (1990) 848-851.

[109] M. A. Jepson, N. L. Simmons, D. T. O'Hagan, B. H. Hirst, Comparison of poly(D,L-lactide-*co*-glycolide) and polystyrene microsphere targeting to intestinal M cells, J. Drug. Target. 1 (1993) 245-249.

[110] A. T. Florence, A. M. Hillery, N. Hussain, P. U. Jani, Nanoparticles as carriers for oral peptide absorption: studies on particle uptake and fate, J. Control. Release 36 (1995) 39-46.

[111] A. M. Hillery, A. T. Florence, The effect of adsorbed poloxamer 188 and 407 surfactants on the intestinal uptake of 60-nm polystyrene particles after oral administration in the rat, Int. J. Pharm. 132 (1996) 123-130.

Chapitre V

[112] J. Seifert, B. Haraszti, W. Sass, The influence of age and particle number on absorption of polystyrene particles from rat gut, J. Anat. 189 (1996) 483-486.

[113] D. T. O'Hagan, The intestinal uptake of particles and the implications for drug and antigen delivery, J. Anat. 189 (Pt 3) (1996) 477-482.

[114] J. Kreuter, Peroral administration of nanoparticles, Adv. Drug Deliv. Rev. 7 (1991) 71-86.

[115] N. Foster, M. Ann Clark, M. A. Jepson, B. H. Hirst, *Ulex europaeus* 1 lectin targets microspheres to mouse Peyer's patch M-cells *in vivo*, Vaccine 16 (1998) 536-541.

[116] M. W. Smith, N. W. Thomas, P. G. Jenkins, N. G. A. Miller, D. Cremaschi, C. Porta, Selective transport of microparticles across Peyer's patch follicle-associated M cells from mice and rats, Exp. Physiol. 80 (1995) 735-744.

[117] C. Porta, P. S. James, A. D. Phillips, T. C. Savidge, M. W. Smith, D. Cremaschi, Confocal analysis of fluorescent bead uptake by mouse Peyer's patch follicle-associated M cells, Exp. Physiol. 77 (1992) 929-932.

[118] J. Pappo, T. H. Ermak, H. J. Steger, Monoclonal antibody-directed targeting of fluorescent polystyrene microspheres to Peyer's patch M cells, Immunology 73 (1991) 277-280.

[119] J. H. Easson, E. Haltner, C. M. Lehr, Bacterial invasion factors and lectins as second-generation bioadhesives, in: E. Mathiowitz, D. E. Chickering, C. M. Lehr (Eds.), Bioadhesion Drug Delivery Systems - Fundamentals, Novel Approaches, and Development, Marcel Dekker, Inc., New York, U.S.A.,1st ed, 1999, pp. 409-431.

[120] A. Pusztai, S. Bardocz, W. B. S. Ewen, Plant lectins for oral drug delivery to different parts of the gastrointestinal tract, in: E. Mathiowitz, D. E. Chickering, C. M. Lehr (Eds.), Bioadhesive Drug Delivery Systems - Fundamentals, Novel Approaches, and Development, Marcel Dekker, Inc., New York, U.S.A., 1st ed, 1999, pp. 387-407.

[121] N. Hussain, P. U. Jani, A. T. Florence, Enhanced oral uptake of tomato lectin-conjugated nanoparticles in the rat, Pharm. Res. 14 (1997) 613-618.

[122] E. Haltner, J. H. Easson, C. M. Lehr, Lectins and bacterial invasion factors for controlling endo- and transcytosis of bioadhesive drug carrier systems, Eur. J. Pharm. Biopharm. 44 (1997) 3-13.

172

[123] P. Arbos, M. A. Campanero, M. A. Arangoa, J. M. Irache, Nanoparticles with specific bioadhesive properties to circumvent the pre-systemic degradation of fluorinated pyrimidines, J. Control. Release 96 (2004) 55-65.

[124] N. Hussain, A. T. Florence, Utilizing bacterial mechanisms of epithelial cell entry: invasin-induced oral uptake of latex nanoparticles, Pharm. Res. 15 (1998) 153-156.

[125] G. J. Russell-Jones, L. Arthur, H. Walker, Vitamin B12-mediated transport of nanoparticles across Caco-2 cells, Int. J. Pharm. 179 (1999) 247-255.

[126] G. J. Russell-Jones, The potential use of receptor-mediated endocytosis for oral drug delivery, Adv. Drug Deliv. Rev. 46 (2001) 59-73.

[127] B. Carreno-Gomez, J. F. Woodley, A. T. Florence, Studies on the uptake of tomato lectin nanoparticles in everted gut sacs, Int. J. Pharm. 183 (1999) 7-11.

[128] M. A. Conway, L. Madrigal-Estebas, S. McClean, D. J. Brayden, K. H. G. Mills, Protection against *Bordetella pertussis* infection following parenteral or oral immunization with antigens entrapped in biodegradable particles: effect of formulation and route of immunization on induction of Th1 and Th2 cells, Vaccine 19 (2001) 1940-1950.

[129] D. H. Jones, S. Corris, S. McDonald, J. C. S. Clegg, G. H. Farrar, Poly(D,L-lactide-*co*-glycolide)-encapsulated plasmid DNA elicits systemic and mucosal antibody responses to encoded protein after oral administration, Vaccine 15 (1997) 814-817.

[130] K. Roy, H. Q. Mao, S. K. Huang, K. W. Leong, Oral gene delivery with chitosan-DNA nanoparticles generates immunologic protection in a murine model of peanut allergy, Nat. Med. 5 (1999) 387-391.

[131] S. J. Challacombe, D. Rahman, H. Jeffery, S. S. Davis, D. T. O'Hagan, Enhanced secretory IgA and systemic IgG antibody responses after oral immunization with biodegradable microparticles containing antigen, Immunology 76 (1992) 164-168.

[132] D. T. O'Hagan, J. P. McGee, J. Holmgren, A. M. Mowat, A. M. Donachie, K. H. G. Mills, W. Gaisford, D. Rahman, S. J. Challacombe, Biodegradable microparticles for oral immunization, Vaccine 11 (1993) 149-154.

[133] D. T. O'Hagan, D. Rahman, H. Jeffery, S. Sharif, S. J. Challacombe, Controlled release microparticles for oral immunization, Int. J. Pharm. 108 (1994) 133-139.

Chapitre V

[134]   S. J. Challacombe, D. Rahman, D. T. O'Hagan,   Salivary, gut, vaginal and nasal antibody responses after oral immunization with biodegradable microparticles, Vaccine 15 (1997) 169-175.

[135]   K. J. Maloy, A. M. Donachie, D. T. O'Hagan, A. M. Mowat, Induction of mucosal and systemic immune responses by immunization with ovalbumin entrapped in poly(lactide-co-glycolide) microparticles, Immunology 81 (1994) 661-667.

[136]   T. Jung, W. Kamm, A. Breitenbach, K. D. Hungerer, E. Hundt, T. Kissel, Tetanus toxoid loaded nanoparticles from sulfobutylated poly(vinyl alcohol)-graft-poly(lactide-co-glycolide): evaluation of antibody response after oral and nasal application in mice, Pharm. Res. 18 (2001) 352-360.

[137]   D. T. O'Hagan, J. P. McGee, M. Lindblad, J. Holmgren,   Cholera toxin B subunit (CTB) entrapped in microparticles shows comparable immunogenicity to CTB mixed with whole cholera toxin following oral immunization, Int. J. Pharm. 119 (1995) 251-255.

[138]   D. T. O'Hagan, K. J. Palin, S. S. Davis,   Poly(butyl-2-cyanoacrylate) particles as adjuvants for oral immunization, Vaccine 7 (1989) 213-216.

[139]   M. Conway, J. Eyles, H. O. Alpar,   Systemic and local immune responses following oral and nasal delivery of microspheres of different sizes, J. Pharm. Pharmacol. 49 (1997) 30.

[140]   I. Gutierro, R. M. Hernandez, M. Igartua, A. R. Gascon, J. L. Pedraz,   Influence of dose and immunization route on the serum Ig G antibody response to BSA loaded PLGA microspheres, Vaccine 20 (2002) 2181-2190.

[141]   D. H. Jones, B. W. McBride, C. Thornton, D. T. O'Hagan, A. Robinson, G. H. Farrar,   Orally administered microencapsulated *Bordetella pertussis* fimbriae protect mice from *B. pertussis* respiratory infection, Infect. Immun. 64 (1996) 489-494.

[142]   M. Murillo, M. J. Grillo, J. Rene, C. M. Marin, M. Barberan, M. M. Goni, J. M. Blasco, J. M. Irache, C. Gamazo, A *Brucella ovis* antigenic complex bearing poly-[ε]-caprolactone microparticles confer protection against experimental brucellosis in mice, Vaccine 19 (2001) 4099-4106.

[143] P. Johansen, F. Estevez, R. Zurbriggen, H. P. Merkle, R. Gluck, G. Corradin, B. Gander, Towards clinical testing of a single-administration tetanus vaccine based on PLA/PLGA microspheres, Vaccine 19 (2000) 1047-1054.

[144] S. C. Chen, D. H. Jones, E. F. Fynan, G. H. Farrar, J. C. Clegg, H. B. Greenberg, J. E. Herrmann, Protective immunity induced by oral immunization with a rotavirus DNA vaccine encapsulated in microparticles, J. Virol. 72 (1998) 5757-5761.

[145] J. E. Herrmann, S. C. Chen, D. H. Jones, A. Tinsley-Bown, E. F. Fynan, H. B. Greenberg, G. H. Farrar, Immune responses and protection obtained by oral immunization with rotavirus VP4 and VP7 DNA vaccines encapsulated in microparticles, Virology 259 (1999) 148-153.

[146] M. Koping-Hoggard, G. Ocklind, H. Guan, B. Jansson, P. Artursson, Chitosan and PEI-pDNA polyplexes: *In vivo* gene expression after tracheal, nasal and oral administration to mice, 1999, pp. 795-796.

RÉSUMÉ ET CONCLUSIONS

RÉSUMÉ ET CONCLUSIONS

Les nanoparticules à base de polymère offrent la possibilité d'administrer des principes actifs par les voies mucosale, orale ou parentérale. C'est ainsi que ces dernières années, de nombreuses molécules actives ont été encapsulées dans ces vecteurs en vue d'améliorer leur activité thérapeutique ou de réduire leurs effets secondaires. Or, si plusieurs méthodes ont été proposées pour la fabrication de ces colloïdes, les études comparant de telles techniques font généralement défaut dans la littérature.

Le but principal de ce travail de thèse a donc été de comparer, du point de vue pharmaceutique et technologique (Chapitres II-III), trois des principales méthodes utilisées dans la préparation des nanoparticules de polymères : l'émulsification-diffusion, le relargage (*salting-out*) et la nanoprécipitation. Afin d'évaluer l'effet de la procédure de préparation sur les caractéristiques des nanoparticules, l'étude a été réalisée en utilisant des formulations standards composées des mêmes matières premières. L'Eudragit® L100-55, un copolymère de l'acide méthacrylique, a été choisi comme polymère constituant de la matrice des nanoparticules tandis que le poly(alcool de vinyle) (PVAL) a servi comme agent émulsifiant. L'ibuprofène, molécule légèrement soluble dans l'eau, a été sélectionné comme principe actif modèle. Dans ce contexte, nous avons d'abord étudié les paramètres physico-chimiques associés à la formation des nanoparticules. Ensuite, les techniques ont été évaluées en fonction de leur capacité à incorporer l'ibuprofène dans ces colloïdes. Enfin, nous avons effectué une approche technologique sur la transposition d'échelle de ces trois procédés de fabrication de nanoparticules.

177

Résumé et conclusions

De même, ce résumé fait le point sur les expériences réalisées avec deux nouvelles entités chimiques possédant une activité anticancéreuse (Chapitre IV). Ces molécules, notamment le DIMATE et le MATE, appartiennent au groupe des inhibiteurs de l'enzyme aldéhyde hydrogénasse (ALDH1). La technique d'émulsification-évaporation, récemment développée et brevetée par notre laboratoire, a été utilisée pour encapsuler ces substances. Les résultats préliminaires concernant l'évaluation biologique *in vitro* des nanoparticules obtenues sont également discutés.

Finalement, les Chapitres I et V ne sont pas repris ici car ce sont des revues de la littérature. Le Chapitre I sert de partie introductive de la thèse et contient une description générale des méthodes les plus utilisées pour la fabrication des nanoparticules à base de polymères préformés. Quant au Chapitre V, il présente une compilation et une discussion des diverses études consacrées à l'application *in vivo* des nanoparticules par voie orale.

CHAPITRE II

Dans la première étape de ce travail de thèse, nous avons évalué la capacité des trois méthodes à encapsuler efficacement un principe actif, l'ibuprofène, qui est un acide faible légèrement soluble dans l'eau. Les méthodes de relargage et d'émulsification-diffusion ont abouti à des nanoparticules chargées en ibuprofène avec des tailles de 140 à 650 nm. L'efficacité d'encapsulation de l'ibuprofène a été améliorée en ajustant le pH de la phase aqueuse utilisée dans la préparation des nanoparticules ainsi que celui du milieu utilisé dans leur purification. Une acidification réduit la solubilité de l'ibuprofène dans l'eau et, en conséquence, limite sa migration vers la phase aqueuse externe. Nous avons aussi constaté que le degré d'incorporation de l'ibuprofène s'accroît avec la taille des nanoparticules. En raison de leur plus grande surface spécifique, les plus petits globules de l'émulsion précurseur ont tendance à perdre davantage d'ibuprofène dans la phase aqueuse externe pendant les étapes de diffusion et de dilution.

Ensuite, une comparaison des nanoparticules de même taille montre que celles préparées par la méthode de relargage présentent des taux de chargement en ibuprofène plus élevés que celles fabriquées par émulsification-diffusion. En effet, plusieurs paramètres intrinsèques de la méthode de relargage favorisent la vitesse de précipitation du polymère ainsi que la vitesse de diffusion du solvant, ce qui conduit à augmenter l'incorporation de l'ibuprofène dans les nanoparticules. Parmi ces paramètres, on peut mentionner la solubilité inférieure de l'Eudragit® L100-55 dans l'acétone, la miscibilité totale de l'acétone avec l'eau et le volume d'eau inférieur utilisé pour la diffusion du solvant dans la technique de relargage. Il faut également noter que les coefficients de diffusion du solvant dans l'eau, calculés à partir de l'équation de Tyn et Calus, ont confirmé partiellement cette hypothèse. Les valeurs des coefficients correspondent à $1{,}34 \times 10^{-5}$ et $0{,}95 \times 10^{-5}$ cm^2 s^{-1} pour l'acétone et l'alcool benzylique, respectivement. En ce qui concerne la nanoprécipitation, elle aboutit à des nanoparticules très fines (140 nm) et faiblement chargées en ibuprofène. Contrairement à ce qui était prévu, une baisse du pH de la phase aqueuse n'a aucun effet sur l'efficacité d'incorporation de l'ibuprofène. En revanche, l'abaissement du pH affecte radicalement le rendement de la suspension finale de nanoparticules car il induit la précipitation d'une fraction importante de polymère sous forme d'agrégats.

Par ailleurs, l'analyse calorimétrique différentielle a démontré que l'ibuprofène incorporé dans les nanoparticules se présente sous forme amorphe ou dispersé à l'état moléculaire dans la matrice de polymère. Cette conclusion a été tirée du fait que nous avons observé une quasi disparition de l'endotherme de fusion de l'ibuprofène dans les échantillons des nanoparticules fabriquées par les techniques de relargage (ΔH_f = 1,25 mJ/mg) et d'émulsification-diffusion (ΔH_f = 1,30 mJ/mg). Considérant le taux d'encapsulation des nanoparticules, ces enthalpies correspondent respectivement à 3,0 et 2,7 % de l'enthalpie de fusion de l'ibuprofène à l'état pur et cristallin (ΔH_f = 144,16 mJ/mg). Dans le cas des nanoparticules préparées par nanoprécipitation, l'absence de transition endothermique correspondant à l'ibuprofène met plus clairement en évidence l'état amorphe ou dispersé de cette molécule dans le réseau de polymère.

En conclusion, ces trois techniques permettent de préparer une large variété de nanoparticules en termes de taille et d'efficacité d'encapsulation du principe actif. Ceci offre la possibilité de moduler certaines propriétés pharmaceutiques et biologiques de ces vecteurs telles que leur profil de libération du principe actif et comportement bioadhésif, ou même leur ciblage passif. On peut également envisager une forme pharmaceutique contenant plus d'un type de nanoparticules en vue de l'administration simultanée de principes actifs incompatibles ou des particules possédant des profils de libération différents.

CHAPITRE III

Dans cette partie de notre étude nous avons réalisé une approche technologique sur le transfert d'échelle des trois techniques étudiées. La préparation des nanoparticules à l'échelle pilote a été conçue en augmentant 20 fois le volume des lots fabriqués à l'échelle laboratoire. Nous avons examiné l'influence des conditions hydrodynamiques sur les caractéristiques physico-chimiques des nanoparticules, notamment leur taille moyenne, la teneur en ibuprofène et la morphologie. A l'échelle pilote, un accroissement de la vitesse d'agitation pendant l'étape d'émulsification provoque une réduction significative de la taille moyenne des nanoparticules de 557 à 174 nm pour la méthode de relargage et de 562 à 230 nm pour l'émulsification-diffusion. L'augmentation du taux de cisaillement conduit à la formation de globules d'émulsion plus fins produisant ainsi des nanoparticules plus petites. La modélisation du rapport vitesse d'agitation-taille des nanoparticules a été poursuivie à partir d'un modèle fondé sur une loi de puissance simple. Ce modèle, fréquemment appliqué aux dispersions liquide-liquide de l'ordre du micromètre et dont la fraction volumique de phase interne est basse, a montré une bonne corrélation lorsqu'il a été adapté aux systèmes nanoémulsionnés destinés à la préparation de nanoparticules. Nous avons également constaté que la transposition à une échelle supérieure des méthodes de relargage et émulsification-diffusion, en gardant constante la puissance par unité de volume, aboutit à des nanoparticules de tailles moyennes plus petites. De même, les nanoparticules obtenues à l'échelle pilote ont montré des taux d'encapsulation d'ibuprofène plus faibles. En revanche, aucune différence significative n'a été détectée dans les valeurs de PVAL résiduel des nanoparticules préparées aux deux échelles. Finalement, en raison du grand volume d'eau utilisé dans l'étape de diffusion du solvant, la technique d'émulsification-diffusion met en évidence un plus grand nombre de difficultés technologiques pour la mise en œuvre d'un protocole de transfert d'échelle.

Concernant la nanoprécipitation, un système en mode continu a été utilisé pour la préparation de nanoparticules à l'échelle pilote. Cette méthode simple et d'exécution rapide permet la production de lots de volumes très variables, de quelques millilitres à plusieurs litres, en ajustant seulement quelques-uns de paramètres du procédé. De même, nous avons déterminé que le temps global pour la fabrication d'un lot de nanoparticules a été plus court pour la nanoprécipitation par comparaison aux deux autres méthodes. Enfin, on a noté à nouveau que les nanoparticules préparées à l'échelle pilote présentent des tailles moyennes plus basses et des taux d'incorporation d'ibuprofène plus faibles que celles obtenues à l'échelle laboratoire.

On peut conclure que la préparation de nanoparticules par les trois techniques à l'échelle laboratoire a été relativement bien reproduite à l'échelle pilote. Bien que les nanoparticules fabriquées aux deux échelles ont montré des caractéristiques similaires en termes de chargement d'ibuprofène, PVAL résiduel et morphologie, il a été constaté que le processus de transfert d'échelle modifie légèrement les caractéristiques des nanoparticules aboutissant ainsi à des nanoparticules plus petites et avec des chargements en principe actif inférieurs.

CHAPITRE IV

La présente étude est le résultat d'une collaboration avec le Laboratoire d'Immunochimie de la Faculté de Médecine Lyon Sud (France) où Quash et coll. ont conçu et synthétisé une série de nouveaux inhibiteurs de l'enzyme ALDH1. Les études biologiques réalisées avec ce groupe de molécules ont montré que deux d'entre elles, le MATE et le DIMATE, présentaient une activité inhibitrice très intense sur divers types de cellules tumorales. Sur la base de ces résultats prometteurs, le travail a eu comme but le développement et la caractérisation d'une formulation parentérale contenant des nanoparticules chargées en inhibiteurs de l'ALDH1.

La technique d'émulsification-évaporation a été sélectionnée pour la préparation des ces nanoparticules car elle permet, *a priori*, d'incorporer le DIMATE (substance huileuse) et le MATE (solide hydrophobe) dans des nanocapsules et des nanospheres, respectivement. En raison de sa biodégradabilité et sa biocompatibilité, le poly(acide lactique) de masse moléculaire de 12 KDa a été choisi comme le constituant des nanoparticules.

Contrairement à ce qui était attendu, nous avons obtenu des taux d'encapsulation très faibles pour les deux molécules. Dans le cas des nanocapsules chargées en DIMATE (153 nm), une fraction importante du principe actif (80,5 %) a été perdue durant l'étape d'évaporation du solvant. La volatilité de cette substance, inconnue à ce moment-là, a été le facteur limitant de l'encapsulation. Quant aux nanosphères contenant le MATE (128 nm), seuls 29,7 % de la quantité initiale de la molécule ont été incorporés aux nanosphères alors que la fraction restante s'est retrouvée libre dans la phase aqueuse externe de la dispersion brute de nanoparticules. Etant donné qu'aucune trace de la substance à l'état solide n'a pu être mise en évidence dans ce milieu, nous avons envisagé l'existence d'une solution micellaire entre le MATE et le poloxamère présent dans la phase aqueuse. En tenant en compte de la concentration micellaire critique du poloxamère 188 (0,09-0,1 %, m/v, à 25 °C) et de sa concentration dans la dispersion finale de nanoparticules (correspondant à 4,0 %, m/v), une solubilisation de cet agent antitumoral est très probable.

En ce qui concerne les études *in vitro*, la dispersion des nanosphères chargées en MATE a présenté une activité inhibitrice sur les cellules cancéreuses DU145 similaire à celle de la solution alcoolique de référence. Ces résultats sont encourageants car, malgré une faible incorporation de MATE dans les nanoparticules, son activité biologique a pu être conservée. En conséquence, il est attendu qu'en augmentant le taux d'encapsulation du MATE, son activité inhibitrice soit potentialisée.

Diverses stratégies sont proposées en vue d'améliorer l'efficacité d'incorporation des inhibiteurs de l'ALDH1. Dans le cas particulier du DIMATE, une autre technique ne comprenant pas d'étape d'évaporation pourrait être testée. Quant au MATE, les stratégies alternatives incluent la modification du pH de la phase externe, le changement de solvant de la phase organique ou même l'utilisation des autres polymères.

CONCLUSION GENERALE

Les principaux avantages et inconvénients des trois méthodes retenues sont résumés dans le Tableau I. D'une façon générale, on peut conclure que les trois méthodes conviennent pour la fabrication des nanoparticules. Il faut noter que la méthode idéale ne peut être choisie qu'en considérant les propriétés de la substance médicamenteuse et du polymère ainsi que les caractéristiques souhaitées des nanoparticules. De même, le rendement de nanoparticules doit être également pris en compte. Finalement, afin de déterminer de façon plus approfondie l'influence de la méthode de préparation sur les caractéristiques,

Tableau I. Résumé des avantages et point faibles des trois méthodes de préparation de nanoparticules contenant de l'ibuprofène [a].

Paramètre technologique ou pharmaceutique	Méthode de préparation		
	Relargage	Emulsification-diffusion	Nanoprécipitation
Taille moyenne des nanoparticules (nm)	123 – 710	108 – 715	70 – 200
Variables susceptibles de modifier la taille	Concentration d'émulsifiant Concentration en polymère de la phase organique Vitesse d'agitation	Concentration d'émulsifiant Concentration en polymère de la phase organique Vitesse d'agitation	Concentration en polymère et type de solvant de la phase organique
Morphologie des nanoparticules			
Efficacité d'encapsulation du principe actif	Elevée à modérée	Modérée à faible	Faible

Ajustement du pH de la phase aqueuse afin d'améliorer l'encapsulation	Possible	Possible	Effet négatif sur le rendement de nanoparticules
Préparation de nanoparticules sans émulsifiant résiduel	Non faisable	Non faisable	Faisable
Rendement de nanoparticules par quantité de solvant organique (mg / g)	100	170	18
Purification	Nécessaire par filtration tangentielle ou centrifugation	Nécessaire par filtration tangentielle ou centrifugation	Pas toujours nécessaire
Transfert d'échelle	Faisable en mode lots; modélisation possible	Faisable en mode lots, mais mise en œuvre plus élaborée que la technique de relargage; modélisation possible	Faisable en mode continu et mise en œuvre rapide
Temps de préparation d'un lot brut de nanoparticules à l'échelle pilote (min)	300	350	120

[a] Étude effectuée en utilisant, pour les trois techniques, des formulations standards à base des mêmes matières premières : Eudragit® L100-55, poly(alcool de vinyle) et ibuprofène.

propriétés et comportement des nanoparticules, les expériences suivantes sont proposées :

- En recourant à une série de principes actifs possédant des solubilités différentes (par exemple classifiés en fonction de leur δ, il est possible de déterminer quels types de molécules seront les mieux incorporées dans les nanoparticules fabriquées par chacune des techniques.

- Dans le cas de la nanoprécipitation, il serait intéressant de recourir à différents polymères afin de corréler les paramètres $\chi_{\text{polymère-solvant}}$ et $\Delta\delta_{\text{polymère-eau}}$ à la formation ou non de nanoparticules.

- La comparaison des propriétés physico-chimiques (porosité, rugosité, potentiel zéta), pharmaceutiques (profil de libération du principe actif) et biologiques (bioadhésivité) des nanoparticules peut être également envisagée.

- Sur la base des données obtenues à l'échelle pilote et en utilisant des modèles propres au génie des procédés, on peut établir une méthodologie pour réaliser un transfert rationalisé de ces trois méthodes à une échelle supérieure.

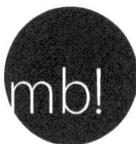

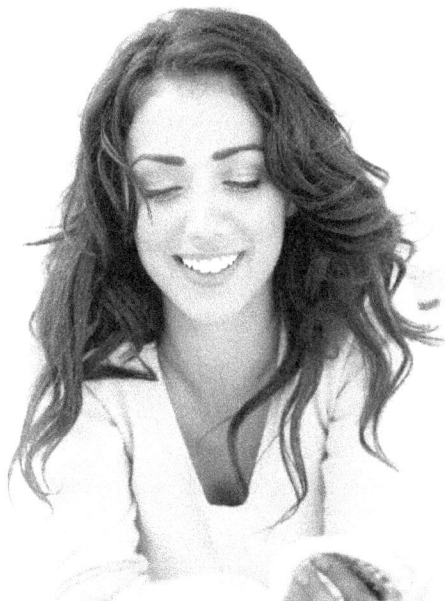

www.ingramcontent.com/pod-product-compliance
Lightning Source LLC
Chambersburg PA
CBHW021046210326
41598CB00016B/1116